Conqu Fibromyalgia

Real Answers and Real Solutions for Real Pain

Michael Lenz, M.D.

ISBN - 9798701786156

Michael Lenz, MD
Board Certified in Pediatrics
Board Certified in Internal Medicine
Diplomat of the American College of Lifestyle Medicine
Diplomat of the Board of Clinical Lipidology
T. Colin Campbell Plant-Based Nutrition Certificate
(262) 513-7500

I dedicate this book to my parents,
John and Lois, who blessed me with their love
both for family and love and care for others.
They modeled love in their marriage to each
other, to their children, and to others.

I also dedicate this to all the patients,
who taught me so much,
by sharing their struggles with me.

Disclaimers and Terms of Use

All readers and users of this content must understand and agree to the following disclaimers and terms of use.

The information presented in this book is provided for informational purposes only. It is NOT intended to be and should NOT be interpreted as medical advice for any medical condition and any individual. It is also not intended to be a substitute for medical advice. The content presented is provided as a starting point in your research and a helpful guide when discussing your individual circumstances with your trusted medical providers. All readers are strongly urged to seek medical attention and guidance regarding any symptoms or health concerns.

The content presented is based on material and sources believed to be accurate and reliable. However, the author, publisher, and any associates, make no representations or warranties with respect to accuracy or completeness.

Any references or links to third parties are for informational purposes only and should not be regarded as endorsements. All readers agree to conduct their own due-diligence research and must assume full responsibility for any outcomes or actions that are experienced after reviewing this content.

Praise for
Conquering Your Fibromyalgia

"Terrific book. I absolutely love it. I have read so many articles on the topic over the years and they often contradict each other or contain inaccurate or incomplete information. Your book exemplifies the kind of doctor you are. You listen to your patients and you have spent countless hours reading and learning about this frustrating disorder.

My endorsement would be:

I have spent countless hours at various types of doctors including chiropractors, OBGYNs, ENTs, Allergists, Physical Therapists, Family Doctors, and Internists attempting to explain my ever-changing symptoms. When I first saw Dr. Lenz a few years ago, his staff spent almost two hours with me asking me countless questions that I did not understand. Eventually, Dr. Lenz came into the room and told me I have Fibromyalgia. After almost 35 years of agonizing pain, unnecessary surgeries, and being told my symptoms were hormone related, I felt like a dignified and respected human again. Thank you, Dr. Lenz for this excellent and comprehensive book. You are the voice for those of us who had none in the medical community for too long.

I love the analogies you use in the book too. General contractor is the perfect way to explain the need for physician training in the area of Fibromyalgia."

Megan F.
Patient of Dr. Lenz

"Love the title and an extremely helpful resource for patients, families, and providers with real world case scenarios and practical tips! Validates the fibromyalgia diagnosis and shares helpful take-home messages. Easy to read and understand, would share with anyone suffering from fibromyalgia type symptoms, their loved ones, and providers."

Heather Toth, MD
Director of the Internal Medicine and
Pediatrics Residency Program
at the Froedtert Medical College of Wisconsin
and Children's Hospital of Wisconsin

~ ~ ~

"This book will provide hope for anyone who is struggling with fibromyalgia. Dr. Michael Lenz provides a comprehensive look at this challenging disease and shares practical tips that can help, highlighting the benefits of a healthful plant-based diet."

Neal Barnard, MD, FACC
President of the Physicians Committee for Responsible Medicine
Adjunct Associate Professor of Medicine at the George Washington
University School of Medicine in Washington, D.C.

Forward

Conquering Your Fibromyalgia is an essential contribution that should be devoured by people who have fibromyalgia and by physicians who treat them. At least four million people in the United States suffer from fibromyalgia (FM), a syndrome encompassing varying and fluctuating levels of pain, fatigue, and sleep disturbances in addition to major difficulties with memory and concentration. There is scant understanding of the condition and certainly no unified approach to treatment. Most people with FM face resistance from skeptical doctors many of whom are convinced that FM is a fictional disorder endorsed by individuals seeking to obtain disability or have other nefarious motivations. Even sympathetic clinicians struggle to find meaningful and long-lasting treatments that improve their patient's sense of well-being and daily functioning.

In his book, Dr. Lenz describes the endless obstacles encountered by many FM patients. This labyrinth needs to be deconstructed as it leads to patient and physician frustration and subjects too many FM sufferers to unnecessary procedures and dangerous medications. A typical example - an individual with complaints of joint pain, chronic fatigue and brain fog initially presents to their primary care physician. After months of various and unsuccessful attempts with non-steroidal anti-inflammatory medications and a few visits to a chiropractor a referral to a specialist is triggered. The rheumatologist might focus solely on the patient's arthritic knee pain and begins a series of steroid injections. More often than not these injections provide transient relief to the joint, but the treatment leaves the patient's vexing problem of fatigue completely unaddressed.

An orthopedic surgeon may be brought in either by the rheumatologist or directly by the frustrated patient. The surgeon pronounces knee damage and may recommend a total knee replacement (TKR). Lenz informs us that in 20 percent of cases, the exasperating pain continues, even after such surgery. The orthopedic surgeon cannot understand the poor outcome: the patient still feels deep discomfort, but the X-rays show a perfectly replaced joint. Physical therapy is consulted, and 12 sessions of hard work does not yield sustained benefit. Increasingly desperate, the physician sends the patient to a pain management expert, who might recommend a muscle relaxer or even opioids—both sedating and potentially addictive drugs which typically cause more problems than they solve. There is still no relief.

A consultation with a psychiatrist occurs next; she might conclude that the panoply of symptoms is a result of the patient's dependency on opiates or underlying anxiety and depression. All too often simply detoxifying the patient or adding an antidepressant does not address the ongoing physical and cognitive complaints. At this point the patient is angry, doctors are contradicting their colleagues, and many clinicians wash their hands and slip away. The patient is left with a greater sense of hopelessness.

Dr Lenz describes this all too familiar scenario,

"For many suffering with FM, they are like an innocent person who has been kidnapped, blindfolded, and tortured by a mysterious and cruel assailant for no apparent reason and with no apparent hope for rescue. Even worse, no one else may believe it is happening because they can't see anything physically wrong with the patient."

Using multiple patient vignettes and colorful analogies to illustrate his important points, Dr. Lenz provides examples of the diagnostic and treatment challenges facing the FM community. Dr. Lenz considers all aspects of the syndrome and offers self-tests for fibromyalgia that can be easily completed. These surveys, when routinely administered, alert the clinician to the possible presence of FM. A working pediatrician and internist, Dr. Lenz offers a unique chapter on children who suffer from this disorder, and whose parents may be told their children have "growing pains" — another variation of "it's not a real problem."

He views the condition throughout the lifespan, a perspective absent from most existing discussions of FM. From this unique clinical vantage point Lenz identifies that FM is often associated with other misunderstood disorders particularly attention deficit/hyperactivity disorder (ADHD) and chronic fatigue syndrome (CFS).

To the reader, Lenz' chapter on attention-deficit/hyperactivity disorder (ADHD) is of particular importance. He notes that these individuals may have an altered response to the pain threshold than others and that childhood ADHD may be a risk factor for FM. Yet, as I have found in my own studies, one of which is cited in this work, their pain is often responsive to stimulant medications for ADHD. The stimulant increases the person's ability to concentrate and at the same time, it decreases their response to pain stimuli. The underlying condition question as to whether ADHD and FM/CFS are two halves of the same walnut is yet to be resolved.

Beyond reviewing the growing literature regarding the use of non-opiate central acting medications for FM, the author endorses a holistic approach combining with exercise, medication, and thoughtful nutrition. Lenz is at his best when describing the role of a plant-based diet in this complement. These are the sections of the book without peril.

Conquering Your Fibromyalgia is a unique addition to the

literature and knowledge about fibromyalgia. I am eager for patients and their providers to integrate this well weaved and highly researched book. Internists, family doctors, and pediatricians, as well as specialists such as rheumatologists, orthopedic surgeons, neurologists, and psychiatrists will be enhanced by the author's mastery.

In years past, depression was often ignored as a "real" problem until finally the medical community acknowledged that this mood disorder is a valid problem affecting million and needs to be treated. Now it is time for physicians to step up and realize fibromyalgia is a similarly debilitating medical problem that strongly merits diagnosis and treatment. Conquering Your Fibromyalgia is an important contribution to bringing both doctors and patients up to speed on this profoundly serious problem today, offering them helpful solutions to their perplexing problem.

Joel Young, MD
Bloomfield Hills, MI
December 2020

Joel L. Young, MD is the Medical Director and Founder of the Rochester Center for Behavioral Medicine. Dr. Young is certified by the American Board of Psychiatry and Neurology with added qualifications in geriatric, forensic, and adolescent psychiatry. He serves as a Clinical Associate Professor of Psychiatry at the Wayne State University School of Medicine. He is also Chief Medical Officer of the Clinical Trials Group of Southeast Michigan. He has served as the primary investigator for more than 70 clinical trials, authoring over 100 articles. He has also authored books on chronic fatigue, mental illness, substance abuse, and ADHD. In addition to clinical care, research, and teaching, Dr. Young also collaborates with the NFL and MLB to evaluate professional athletes.

Table of Contents

Introduction

When I started medical school in 1992, I was oblivious to the diagnosis of fibromyalgia. When I finished medical school in 1996, I was still unaware of this disorder. Despite seeing many patients who likely had fibromyalgia, I was blinded to the diagnosis, let alone how to help the suffering that many patients endured.

The following online testimonial was in response to an article in the New York Times on the use of artificial intelligence for making medical diagnoses. Her story resonates with other stories of my patients and shares common features.

"I would have loved this [artificial intelligence] 25 years ago, before having five painful surgeries for a disease I didn't have. In the past seven years, as symptoms shifted into high gear, I've seen four gynecologists, four orthopedic specialists, two primary care physicians, two physical therapists, two masseurs, two acupuncturists, two pain specialists, one gastroenterologist, one chiropractor, and a Feldenkrais practitioner. That's 21 practitioners who all got it wrong. Can I have my time and cash returned, please? BTW, the right answer is fibromyalgia."

Sadly, her story, and possibly yours, or a loved one's is not unique. While not everyone has all of these problems, and some of you may not even be 25 years old yet, for many people, fibromyalgia is mysterious. Many have pursued potential solutions and wild goose chases only leading to false hopes and frustrations.

There is a big blind spot when it comes to fibromyalgia.

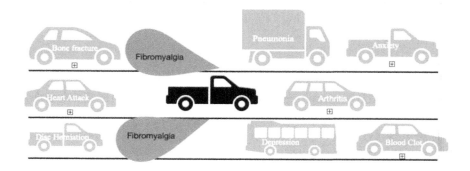

When I was finishing my medical residency in pediatrics and internal medicine in 2000, I started to read about fibromyalgia, a mysterious illness. There was never a grand rounds talk about fibromyalgia. Grand rounds presentations and lectures help doctors and other healthcare professionals to be familiar with the latest advancements, insights, and treatments for a variety of medical conditions. Lectures cover a wide range of medical specialties, so that attendees can learn the latest thought leadership in their specialty as well as in several specialties outside of their own. Most hospitals maintain education departments that arrange lecture programs and provide this continuing medical education. Grand rounds are a significant source of ongoing medical education after medical school and residency.

But, as I will explain, fibromyalgia and fibromyalgia-like syndromes are insidious and pervasive throughout all the specialties. I am sure I saw many patients who had fibromyalgia and chronic pain. Still, I couldn't identify or diagnose something I didn't even know existed. Admittedly, there was a lot to cover in my visits with patients. Diabetes, high cholesterol, smoking addiction, emphysema, high blood pressure, obesity, heart disease, depression, anxiety, asthma, skin disorders, orthopedic injuries, intestinal disorders, headaches, insomnia, and arthritis, among many other conditions were a lot to learn and master.

Identifying the syndromes of fibromyalgia is a challenge for health practitioners. Diagnosis requires a meticulous and careful ear listening for the clues. Medical management requires persistent and caring guidance. There are typically, no easy or quick fixes for this elusive and misunderstood condition.

Is fibromyalgia real?

Many people have either been told or read that fibromyalgia isn't real, or it is just all in their heads, implying that it is just a figment of their imagination. This misunderstanding, unfortunately, causes harm and is a disservice to those suffering. If you are one of the estimated 4 million people in the United States who are suffering from fibromyalgia, then you know it is real. You have probably seen more than one doctor, yet you have not received the help you need to feel better. You were likely dismissed and told that everything is fine. At the same time, you may have been referred to several different specialists. It is also likely that none of these practitioners saw the forest from the trees or detected an overriding increased sensitivity of the nervous system and a decreased ability to inhibit painful sensations.

You may have gone down the path of unfulfilled hopes by well-intentioned medical providers. There may have been a bulge seen on an MRI of your back, yet you continue to have pain despite multiple injections. You may have had MRIs of your brain looking for causes of your headaches or MRIs of your neck looking for causes of your neck pain. You may have had a hysterectomy for chronic pelvic pain or back surgery or knee surgery but still have a significant amount of pain afterward. You may have had foot surgery for a neuroma, and despite multiple surgeries, continue to report much pain.

A lack of awareness, confidence, and comfort with fibromyalgia (FM) is typical for most physicians, and there are likely many reasons for this. One reason is that it doesn't rest on the shoulders of one specialty. Rheumatology may make a diagnosis, but they typically don't manage it. They have enough to cover, caring for those with classic inflammatory diseases like lupus and rheumatoid arthritis. Most pain specialists started their careers in anesthesiology with less face-to-face care. They tend to be more involved in doing procedures instead of a comprehensive approach to treating fibromyalgia. The symptoms of fibromyalgia-like pain intersect with every specialty. The environment of medicine is one where, complex conditions tend to be managed by specialists.

Medicine does a great job at managing acute problems like a heart attack or infectious diseases. Orthopedic procedures to repair damaged bones and joints continue to provide good results. There also is a strong bent to diseases that can be handled with procedures for medical problems like repairing a damaged heart valve. This predominance is somewhat financially driven as the reimbursement for procedures is much higher than cognitive management of chronic non-operative health conditions including fibromyalgia.

Another factor is that most of the medications we have for managing fibromyalgia are off patent. Therefore, the pharmaceutical industry does not push education for off-patent medications compared to new patented biologic agents available to treat diseases. Also, there isn't a single medicine that has been shown to perform as a blockbuster fibromyalgia cure with consistency for most people. This situation often leaves you, the patient, in "no man's land." You might be shuffled from your internist to the rheumatologist who makes the diagnosis but doesn't actively manage the FM. You are then sent back to the family practice or internal medicine physician to manage a disease they don't have the training, understanding, confidence, and comfort in treating adequately. What is needed is a comprehensive, multifaceted approach.

Thankfully, there has been a significant increase in our understanding of FM in the last couple of decades. It routinely takes about 17 years for new medical research to be put into practice. I hope to significantly shorten this delay so that if you are suffering from FM, you don't have to wait any longer to receive the help you need.

This complicated condition could be best managed by an excellent general medical "contractor" with a comprehensive understanding of the disorder. The Canadian guidelines for managing fibromyalgia recommend that the primary care physician become comfortable and take the lead in providing personal 360-degree care. This is similar to the way a general contractor in construction has to have an exceptional understanding of the foundation, concrete, plumbing, electrical, carpentry, drywall, countertops, carpeting, roofing, and landscaping. In medicine, it would be someone who understands all of the organ systems and the interplay in symptoms and can connect the dots to superficially disconnected complaints.

An excellent internist and pediatrician or family practice doctor who is willing to learn and implement such medical knowledge would be well suited for this challenge. It also requires patience, perseverance, coaching, and a desire to motivate and encourage patients as they get through the ups and downs of fibromyalgia. This is the role and commitment I have embraced as a pediatrician and internist, and I find it very rewarding to help those, like you, who have endured FM. My goal is to help lift you out of the "quicksand" you may feel stuck in, because of the misconceptions by many in the medical community.

I started researching FM in the early 2000s and have since grown immensely in my understanding. Further research has enlightened this once misunderstood illness. I continue to see a wide variety of patients with many different medical complaints. Still, many have at their core a "bent" functioning of the pain system. This shift in the nervous system may manifest as diffuse body pain, chronic pain in one part of the body, or a mixture of both, where there is diffuse pain with one area of the body predominating.

I started seeing patterns such as a familial tendency. For example, there may have been a patient's father who had migraines. Now they are suffering from intense menstrual periods. I see patients who may have had irritable bowel syndrome earlier in life and now have developed pain in multiple areas in the body. More and more dots get connected. A picture of a nervous system is revealed that was designed to alert us to bodily injury. Now it is transformed into one that has been bent or shifted to a state of high alert. The pain alarm goes off, signaling an injury is occurring despite no specific or limited damage.

When I was in college, in the dorms, occasionally someone would pull a prank and set off the fire alarm. The fire alarm was so loud and piercing, it was impossible to ignore while waiting for what seemed like a long time for the alarm to be turned off. The wait was very uncomfortable and disruptive and made it virtually impossible to go back to sleep. For someone with fibromyalgia, having a pain alarm go off whether it is moderate, severe, or extreme can completely disrupt your ability to function optimally. As we will learn more about later, a healthy person would perceive the sound as mild noise and not wake up or be bothered by it.

There is a lot of up-to-date information and research shedding new light on our understanding of fibromyalgia-related disorders. There is so much for me to share with you that it can be overwhelming to give and receive this information. But just like a good meal, it is best to consume and digest these insights one bite at a time. There isn't a magic formula, though. My hope, with this book, is to provide you with insight and a more in-depth understanding of what you or your loved one is experiencing. With this understanding, I hope to assist you with this complicated and challenging health issue that can overwhelm and substantially interfere with your ability to function.

This book can be used to complement what you learn at an office visit. It can help educate you as a patient or your loved one who is trying to understand what they have never experienced. One of the treatments for chronic pain is cognitive therapy. This therapy typically involves building a deeper understanding of what you are going through and working on strategies to overcome it. There is only so much information that can be shared in a 15, 30, or 60-minute office visit. There is a lot to take in, and you likely have many questions on the "whys" of fibromyalgia. Hopefully, you can get most of them answered, although there are still many details of FM syndrome to be fleshed out.

Nearly every day, I care for a patient who has some chronic pain or fibromyalgia-like disorder. "You aren't that special," I often say. What I mean is that you are not alone. You endure a disease many others are battling, and there is hope. I have helped many patients suffering from fibromyalgia-like pain and hope the wisdom I have learned along the way can also help you or your loved one. Sharing what I have learned through caring for hundreds of patients may help you understand what you are going through, and there is hope.

I want to educate, inspire, and equip you as you walk through this battle.

Fibromyalgia-like pain syndromes are commonly seen but often not recognized and diagnosed by physicians. There are many reasons for this lack of recognition. Fibromyalgia is where depression was 40 years ago when much of the general public and physicians believed that severely depressed people should try to "get it together." Most physicians at the time did not understand the sheer impossibility of "looking on the bright-side" for someone suffering from depression. Few doctors prescribed antidepressants, although various classes of antidepressants had been available for many years.

Now, moving to the present, many people understand depression is more than a passing mood and accept it as a real disorder that can be treated. On a related note, many with fibromyalgia-related problems have been placed on antidepressants but didn't actually have depression and subsequently didn't respond to this treatment. The symptom of fatigue wasn't from depression but was from fibromyalgia-related problems. So, a walk through this disorder will hopefully do many things.

If you don't have FM, you will, at a minimum, gain a deeper understanding of what you or your loved one is experiencing. If you do have FM, you will feel validated for what you have had to endure. You also will receive actionable steps you can take to thrive, not just survive with FM and its related disorders. In addition, you can get a 360-degree understanding of what FM is. You can then learn practical and realistic strategies for tackling it. You will learn not just about medications that can help treat fibromyalgia but also the roles of stress and lifestyle on the management of fibromyalgia. You will understand more about how to effectively use exercise to manage symptoms. You also will gain greater insight into the role a whole-foods plant-based (WFPB) diet can have in reducing symptoms of fibromyalgia and fibromyalgia related disorders.

Section One

Chapter 1
The "Buy-In"
Inform, Inspire, and Equip

What is a buy-in? If you are coaching a team, you need to get buy-in from the team to have alignment with the mission. But the winning for the person with fibromyalgia (FM), is not to win a game but to function better and have more tolerable pain. I sometimes refer to fibromyalgia as the "F" word. In America, that word signifies an expletive and is sometimes how people feel when they are diagnosed with fibromyalgia. It is something that many don't like to hear or say. I have had some nervousness in telling patients they had fibromyalgia and used the word centralized pain syndrome to skirt the stigma and misunderstanding often connected with FM.

The revelation that someone has FM will hit each person at different levels, but your response will impact your recovery. With many chronic diseases like diabetes or heart disease, you aren't the passive receiver of medical therapy but an active participant in your care. There won't be any quick fixes but a combination of approaches to help you manage your health the best. If you are someone who initially is skeptical, I ask you to take the time to digest it all and let it simmer. Write down questions or take notes on areas that resonate, especially with you or your loved one.

Every person's story is unique, and not everything may thoroughly apply to you, but many of the general principles likely will. Your past experiences and explanations for the problems you face have to be filtered through. You may have been through several, even a dozen doctors, surgeries, and injections without much long-lasting relief. This understanding may also hit at a deeper existential reality. Do our perceptions of reality determine truth or has something been skewed?

When a new coach takes over responsibilities for coaching the team, for the team to be successful, the players will need to buy-in to the philosophy of the new coach. They also need to trust that his plan for the team will be successful both for each player individually and as a whole team collectively. Sometimes this goes well, and other times it doesn't. A coach can layout the new offensive scheme they will be running, the background on how it works, and why it works. He can also put together an excellent practice plan to teach them and give workouts that the team should do in the off-season to improve their skills and get stronger. However, the individual players need to trust in the coach. If they don't, it can lead to poor performance for the team. They have to implement offensive and defensive schemes.

When I played football in high school, we ran the Wishbone offense and did pretty well but could not win the conference championship. My coach, who was also my chemistry teacher, would say that it is not the offense but the execution. His point applies to the management of FM. The coach doesn't run the plays but teaches, directs, guides, and calls the plays and helps to get the most out of each individual's talent. I am hoping in a way, to be your coach, taking extra time to explain the reasoning behind your struggles. I would love to take the time with each of my patients struggling with fibromyalgia-related disorders to share what is in this book, but there is so much to cover. This realization inspired me to write this book.

The information on fibromyalgia may be a new concept and run counter to what you may have told about your symptoms of pain by other physicians you have seen over the years. Learning what fibromyalgia is sometimes and, to some extent, can be hard to accept. However, seeing how all the dots connect is very eye-opening. It is important to have a "beginner's mind." It can be bittersweet. The sweetness is understanding what you have and getting better. The bitterness is considering the "what ifs?" "What if I would have gotten properly diagnosed and treated in childhood or early adulthood when I first had symptoms?"

Get engaged. The engaged healthcare consumer is one who is active in the management of their health. Embrace fibromyalgia and what it is and get involved in the therapies to treat it and avoid those that aggravate it. If you have questions, write them down. Keep track of your activity level. One example is getting an activity monitor to track your steps and then pace yourself. More treatment options will be discussed in subsequent chapters.

There is an existential challenge you might face, to some extent, as we have been told to trust our feelings. Still, with fibromyalgia, our perceptions or sensations don't represent the whole of the physical reality. Someone may not have anything that is causing tissue damage, or if they do, it is smaller than one would expect from the degree of pain being experienced. There has to be an acceptance of the concept of fibromyalgia and the plan to help make it better. In this book, you'll gain a deeper understanding of fibromyalgia and ways to help manage it better. Be prepared to be informed, inspired, and equipped. Every story is unique. My goal for this book is to help inform you, inspire you, and equip you to control your fibromyalgia.

Let's look at "Jane's" story.

"Jane" is a woman in her 40s whose story may resonate with you. Her first significant problems started after she was in a car accident in her 20s, after which she developed persistent neck pain. Before

that, Jane had relatively minor issues with pain that only briefly disrupted her life. The only significant pain she did suffer were painful menstrual periods in high school at times and some occasional headaches. Digging more in-depth, she did report a history of growing pains in her legs at night during sleep that came and went based on how physically active she was in high school. On further discussion and evaluation, she was found to have restless leg syndrome, a very treatable medical condition. She recalls that the more active she was, the less intense her restless leg symptoms were. She was an athlete until late high school and remained very physically active overall, working out on an almost daily basis.

After the accident, however, her activity level markedly decreased. Her pain level went up despite the doctors telling her months after the car crash that she had healed well and should be on to a good recovery. She had been given ibuprofen and Tylenol, which didn't help much. She was placed on Vicodin, but it didn't cure her, and she continued to be in moderate to severe pain. Her chronic neck pain persisted for years. The pain worsened to the point where the doctor she had been seeing referred her to pain management. Along the way, she had MRIs of her back and neck, showing some disc bulging. She received injections without any significant long-term benefit. Opiates were used, but this seemed only to worsen the pain and required escalating doses to manage it.

I had a chance to see her and took a careful history, physical exam, and screening blood work. I used the fibromyalgia criteria to make the diagnosis of FM and then began treatment. Restless leg syndrome is a problem that can wreak havoc on fibromyalgia if untreated. As with many who have restless leg syndrome and fibromyalgia, she also had untreated ADHD which also was discovered through a careful history and use of the World Health Organization adult ADHD questionnaire. She had a high IQ and had graduated from college but struggled with adult ADHD without knowing it.

The first step was to look at the playing field and see what she faced.

I took the time to explain what fibromyalgia was and how there also was a connection with the other frustrations she had endured. We started with treating her restless leg syndrome. A good night's sleep is crucial for treating fibromyalgia. She was placed on gabapentin, and the dose was adjusted so she could fall and stay asleep without feeling drowsy in the morning. She noticed a dramatic improvement in how rested she felt in the AM. Then we were able to address her previously undiagnosed and untreated ADHD. Under treatment with Adderall XR, she discovered that she no longer felt overwhelmed and could get through her day at work and home and didn't feel overwhelmed. In the past, she had noticed how stress seemed to cause more pain.

Stress for her and many with fibromyalgia was the feeling of being overwhelmed, but now she could do what I like to call TCB, taking care of business. She was able to complete tasks and get through the daily grind. The repetitive details that in the past were very challenging were done with relative ease. She was able to accomplish her tasks. Jane also noticed that she wasn't feeling as much pain and had a lot more energy.

Her "brain fog" also seemed to be lifted. Her FIQR (Fibromyalgia Impact Questionnaire Revised) score, a comprehensive measure of overall fibromyalgia difficulties, dropped from a very high range down to a moderate level. She was placed on a low dose of duloxetine, a medicine that can help decrease the intensity of pain by increasing her low levels of the neuro-transmitters serotonin and norepinephrine. Also, she was gradually becoming more active. She remembers having been active until the accident and felt her best, but after the accident, she became the most sedentary she had ever been in her life. She went from getting 15,000 steps a day on average to about 2,000 steps a day. But now she gradually became more active. She increased her activity throughout the day and kept track of her steps on her activity counter. Each week she increased her levels carefully by about 10%. We discussed how rapid increases in her activity were likely to backfire. She also had more time to exercise. She was more efficient in accomplishing her tasks because *her ADHD was now treated. In the past, even when she could muster up the energy to do some exercise, she had always felt guilty because she had so much unfinished business from staying late at work, having to take some home to finish later, or having to care for her house and children.*

She had also struggled with her weight, which had added to her frustration. She had gained 100 lbs. since the accident ten years prior and felt disappointed in how she "let herself go." She knew that her current "SAD" (standard American diet) wasn't healthy, but when she felt stressed, she craved the calorie-dense, nutritionally depleted food. I discussed how food choices could have a significant impact on fibromyalgia. It was also understandable given she had fallen into the trap so many in her situation suffer. She had failed so many attempts before to lose weight only for her will power to give out as she regained all the weight and more.

We discussed trying a low-fat whole-food plant-based diet and how it could help her feel better and lose weight. She understood that eating a diet full of whole grains, fruits, vegetables, beans, and a small number of nuts and seeds with spices was healthy, but she felt overwhelmed in learning how to navigate this new way of eating. She agreed and went through a program with a dietitian, teaching her how to eat this entirely new way. She started gradually by substituting a healthy breakfast with oatmeal and fruit instead of her typical sausage, eggs, and a buttered muffin or a quick donut with coffee and cream. The second week, she started adding a healthy lunch, and the third week she had added dinner. She noticed that her bloating that was so normal to her that she previously hadn't even brought it up to me completely went away. Her long-standing constipation faded.

During this process, she was weaned off opioids as well. After three months, she felt like she had her life back. She never realized that she could feel that good. She had lost about 15 lbs. and was more vigorous. Her FIQR score, a broad measure of fibromyalgia suffering, went to 15, a healthy rating, down from her very high score of 77 she had when I first met her.

Jane didn't get better in one day. It took months. If you have fibromyalgia and this story resonates with you or someone you know, be inspired and have hope that you too, can get through this with time.

What is Fibromyalgia?

Fibromyalgia is a chronic disorder characterized by widespread and persistent non-inflammatory musculoskeletal pain. The area in the brain where pain is experienced is more sensitive, known as central pain sensitization. Pain is experienced when there is either tissue damage or perceived tissue damage. A simple metaphor is a fire alarm. The alarm is designed to go off when there is a fire, but the alarms in those with fibromyalgia go off when the temperature in the room rises, but there is no fire. Additional symptoms usually include fatigue, insomnia, morning stiffness, depression, anxiety, and cognitive problems such as forgetfulness, concentration difficulties, mental slowness, memory and attention problems.

Furthermore, the majority of FM patients usually have a predisposition to experience negative moods including anger, anxiety, self-consciousness, irritability, emotional instability, and depression. They commonly respond poorly to environmental stress, interpret ordinary situations as threatening, and can experience minor frustrations as hopelessly overwhelming. They have an impaired health-related quality of life. There are higher levels of catastrophizing.

Fibromyalgia has been a medical mystery for a long time. Extensive research has been unraveling this mysterious syndrome over the last couple of decades. Through the mist, a solid understanding of fibromyalgia is being revealed. Some factors are known to predispose individuals to FM such as genes, lifestyle, and physical trauma. One of the most accepted hypotheses regarding FM is the presence of central sensitization to pain and deficits in endogenous, built in, pain inhibitory processes. There is strong scientific evidence to support these observations. Evidence supporting this includes low thresholds and tolerance of pain, known as hyperalgesia and allodynia that characterize fibromyalgia. Tissue damage is felt more intensely and things that do not cause tissue damage are experienced as pain. Experiments that measure pain sensitization at different levels of stimuli show greater responses in areas of the brain that process pain in those with FM in comparison to healthy individuals.

Fibromyalgia is also characterized by abnormal somatosensory processing stemming from changes within the central nervous system, i.e., brain and spinal cord. It can also be thought of as an imbalance between excitatory and inhibitory influences on the central nervous system's pain-management pathways. There has been a change or shift in how the brain and spinal cord "listen" to the body. It has nothing to do with damage to the muscles and structures supporting them, as the name implies. The small differences in mitochondria of the muscles in those with FM is likely related to deconditioning and can be changed with a graduated exercise program and healthy diet. It is not a cause but a downstream result.

The name was given before we had the current insight and understanding of fibromyalgia. This misnomer in the early observations of the syndrome is similar to malaria. Malaria was thought initially by the Romans to be caused by breathing in the "bad air" of swamp gas. It wasn't until the invention of the microscope that it was discovered that the parasite from infected mosquitos was the cause. Also, FM is a syndrome. A syndrome is a collection of signs and symptoms, but the underlying cause is often not understood initially. Before the cause of AIDS (Acquired Immune Deficiency Syndrome) was discovered, we knew something was acquired that weakened the immune system. The opportunistic infections and cancers observed were used to describe the syndrome. It is more often called HIV disease now as powerful antiviral medications suppress the levels of HIV. Hence, AIDS is very rare compared to when I was in medical school and residency in the early and mid-1990s.

What is the "microscope" unveiling the cause of FM?

Functional MRI imaging has revealed what was once hidden. The brain's areas used to assess pain light up at lower pressures during experiments applying pressure to the thumb. For example, functional MRI studies showed that the brains in those with FM process the lower pressure the same as if the thumb is being injured at high pressures in a person unaffected by FM. Those who are unaffected require 2-3 times the levels of pressure to activate the same brain area involved in pain perception. There is also MRI spectroscopy showing insights into the tissue content of the brain and has demonstrated differences. There are reductions in the functions of parts of the brain known as the anterior cingulate cortex, which is very involved in pain, executive function, and autonomic control.

Low levels of dopamine are associated with restless legs, ADHD, and "fibro fog." Reduced dopamine synthesis is found in some regions of the brainstem, thalamus, and limbic system. The areas are those involved in cognitive function, pain control, movement (stiffness), and autonomic function (think stress). The areas of the insular cortex were strongly matched to the clinical pain.

Take home message:
Fibromyalgia is real and involves differences in how the brain and spinal cord process and listen to the body.

What are the features of FM syndrome?

Fibromyalgia syndrome includes problems with heightened pain sensitivities known as central pain. Those with FM feel pain more intensely with the same pressure or peripheral nerve stimulation than those without fibromyalgia (FM). There are also cognitive problems known as "fibro fog," which include difficulties with attention, focus, and initiating activities, among other challenges. There are also problems with sleeping. Each of these issues is observed, but the medical community has not consistently made the underlying connections to the causes very well. This difficulty is likely due to a combination of factors, including a highly specialized medical community and a lack of training for physicians on FM and associated problems.

Why do you want to know what causes fibromyalgia?

You want to understand it because it is very frustrating living with it. And to be honest, it is very disappointing for most doctors to treat. When a typical doctor has a patient with FM-like syndrome on the schedule, they may cringe a little and have to take a deep breath. You report to the doctor the different areas of your body where you have problems. The testing doesn't show any issues such as a thyroid problem, anemia, heart failure, or inflammatory disease. Both you and the doctor have been trying to navigate through this. You have been to many specialists, tried supplements, and tried alternative therapies with limited success.

What's different about FM compared to other health conditions?

Other illnesses often go away quickly with treatment, while FM does not. Tackling an infection or appendicitis is relatively easy once the diagnosis is made. FM is not that way. It is much more complicated. For those with fibromyalgia, it has not been a simple, easy fix. All the simple, easy remedies such as using acetaminophen or ibuprofen for tension headaches or painful periods have likely been used for months or years before someone even seeks medical advice. They may have offered some relief, but over time the pain has only worsened. So, let's dig into the details.

Fibromyalgia is a disorder characterized by widespread musculoskeletal pain accompanied by fatigue, sleep, memory, and mood issues. Researchers believe that fibromyalgia amplifies painful sensations by affecting the way your brain processes pain signals. Fibromyalgia syndrome (FMS) is now a recognized clinical entity causing chronic and disabling pain. For several centuries, muscle pains have been known as rheumatism and then as muscular rheumatism.

In 1592, in the book "*Liber de reumatismo*," Guillaume deBaillou described some muscular pains similar to FM. This is probably the very first medical description of FM. An important step was made by William Balfour, a surgeon in Edinburgh who was the first, in 1815, to describe "a special pain, usually driven by an inflammatory action, involving fibrous and white tissues, belonging to muscles and joints, like tendons, aponeurosis." He called this widespread pain "fibrositis."

In 1880, a U.S. psychologist named George M Beard wrote about a collection of symptoms consisting of fatigue, widespread pain, and psychological disturbances. He called it 'neurasthenia' and attributed the problems to the stress of modern life. For many years, lack of a unifying etiology and a universal terminology hindered the understanding and recognition of FM.

In 1904, a pathologist, Ralph Stockman, reported evidence of inflammatory changes occurring in the fibrous, intramuscular septa of biopsies from afflicted patients. That finding led Sir William Gowers to introduce the term "fibrositis" to describe the inflammation of fibrous tissue in his description of lower back pain. In subsequent years, the terms fibrositis, fibromyositis, psychogenic, psychosomatic, or muscular rheumatism have all been used as descriptors for this syndrome.

The term fibrositis was coined by Gowers in 1904 and was not changed to fibromyalgia until 1976. Smythe laid the foundation of modern FM syndrome in 1972 by describing widespread pain and tender points. The first controlled clinical study with validation of known symptoms and tender points was published in 1981. This same study also proposed the first data-based criteria. The critical concept that FM and other similar conditions are interconnected was introduced in 1984.

The first American College of Rheumatology criteria for FM were published in 1990, and neurological and hormonal mechanisms with central sensitization were developed in the 1990s. Serotonergic/norepinephrine drugs were first shown to be effective in 1986. Initial criteria for FM required having 11 or more tender points of the 18 typical trigger points in the body, but the updated guidelines in 2016 no longer require it. We recognize that fibromyalgia is on a spectrum both within the individual and from person to person. Symptoms are not the same every day or every part or every time of each day.

Patients with fibromyalgia have chronic (>3 months) pain that is generalized, occurs in multiple sites, and is associated with fatigue, sleep problems, and cognitive or somatic symptoms. A chief complaint of "I hurt all over" should alert the doctor and the patient to a possible diagnosis of fibromyalgia. A recent patient described it like having the flu with diffuse muscle and joint aches. However, there are no fevers, chills, or sweats. Pain may be generalized initially or more often localized to a specific site or region, such as the lower back or neck. The diagnosis may be missed when a broader pain history is not considered in the evaluation of seemingly isolated symptoms.

It is somewhat analogous to a teacher having a challenging classroom to teach. There may be a particular child who is very disruptive and gets noticed. There may be a few other students who are also causing problems but not as severe, so they don't draw the same level of attention. Chronic back pain may be the chief complaint, but other areas of the body are painful as well but less intense. A body diagram or checklist indicating where you have had any areas of chronic pain, tightness, soreness, or achiness type symptoms can help in diagnosis. The new criteria for FM involve counting the number of locations in the body where someone has pain. The higher number of areas of pain indicate worse fibromyalgia.

Fibromyalgia is a common problem affecting many people to some degree. There has been a profound misunderstanding of what fibromyalgia is. For years, many denied its existence. This viewpoint is likely related to a lack of understanding of this complicated disorder. Many patients would have been told that they are hypochondriacs or worse: that they are faking it. Even if they weren't told they were faking it, their perception was that the doctor believed they were.

The good news is that much has been learned in the last 10 to 15 years to better understand this often-frustrating disease. I finished my medical residency in internal medicine and pediatrics in the year 2000. At that time, there was a vague understanding of what it was and how best to treat it. It had never come up with my mentors, in my clinics, during my residency, and I had never heard any talks on fibromyalgia. I had done some research and started to get a grainy understanding of what it was.

Fortunately, research has expanded our understanding. I have continued to grow more and can bring you a better understanding of this complicated disease. Other physicians and medical researchers have devoted much of their medical profession to research in this area on whose shoulders I rest in writing this book. Caring for hundreds of patients with fibromyalgia has taught me invaluable lessons over the years. And, of course, early in my career, I did not understand what I do now.

For many suffering with FM, they are like an innocent person who has been kidnapped, blindfolded, and tortured by a mysterious and cruel assailant for no apparent reason and with no apparent hope for rescue. Even worse, no one else may believe it is happening because they can't see anything physically wrong with them.

For example, you don't have any apparent weakness like someone who had a stroke or multiple sclerosis. You have normal-looking joints, unlike someone who has rheumatoid arthritis. You have a healthy-looking colon and small intestine, unlike one suffering from inflammatory bowel disease or colon cancer. I hope to remove the mask and reveal this mysterious disease to you, with a better understanding, to help guide you to more comfortable living and thriving instead of just surviving.

Fibromyalgia is really on a spectrum. The central nervous system consists of the spinal cord, brain stem, and brain, which can dampen or heighten the sensitivities of the pain experienced. There is a complex interaction of nerves and the signaling between different parts of the brain, brain stem, and spinal cord. This signaling goes back and forth constantly. Peripheral pain is pain caused by problems outside the central nervous system. Peripheral pain generators include mechanical issues like a broken bone or osteoarthritis, and it also includes inflammatory causes such as gout, lupus, and rheumatoid arthritis.

As we walk through this, I hope you can look at some preconceptions most people have about pain. Where do we feel pain? What is the function of pain? There is a continuum of pain perception. There are rare diseases where some people experience little or no pain with injuries and tissue damage. One example is leprosy, where bacteria damage nerves so that one can't feel pain. This lack of awareness can lead to injuries and progressive damage to those injured areas. On the other spectrum are those with severe fibromyalgia who feel the heightened levels of pain with relatively little or no tissue damage.

Most people rightly assume that the location where they feel pain is where their bodies have a mechanical problem such as arthritis or inflammation. A broken toe results in significant pain in that toe because there is an injury there. However, common issues such as osteoarthritis often contain a mixture of both tissue injury and fibromyalgia-like pain. For most with osteoarthritis of the knee, for example, there is some bone swelling from reduced cartilaginous cushioning in the joint. However, there is a considerable difference in pain reported by individuals with the same amount of cartilage loss. How do we know this? Many people have "bone on bone" seen on their x-ray, where there is a nearly complete loss of cartilage. However, they report minimal or no pain.

There also are some people who indicate a considerable amount of pain despite having a relatively healthy-appearing x-ray. About 10 to 20 percent of people still have significant pain after a hip or knee replacement (THA or TKA). In essence, persistent pain is due to what many refer to as fibromyalgia-like pain, also known as central pain amplification. Research has demonstrated that these patients have alterations in central nervous system neurotransmitters that, at least in part, lead to both augmented pain and sensory processing and comorbid symptoms.

Surgical outcomes from joint replacements are affected by presurgical fibromyalgia scores. A study in 2015 by Dr. Daniel Clauw and colleagues demonstrated that for every one-point increase in the fibromyalgia symptom survey score, there was an 18% increase in the odds of failure to meet the threshold of 50% improvement of their hip or knee pain after hip or knee replacement. This finding is important because the estimated lifetime risk of symptomatic knee osteoarthritis is about 45%. Although TKA and THA have been shown to improve chronic pain and function, studies estimate that about 20% of knee replacement and 10% of hip replacement patients fail to derive the desired analgesic benefit. Every one-point increase in the fibromyalgia survey score from 0 to 31 was associated with consuming an adjusted 9 mg more oral morphine equivalents to treat postoperative pain following THA and TKA. The Widespread pain index is shown in Chapter 5 and is part of the diagnostic criteria for FM.

Examples of cognitive problems include trouble concentrating, forgetfulness, and disorganized or slow thinking. Cognitive problems are increasingly recognized as a major feature of FM, with dysfunction being seen in working memory and executive function. Self-reported questionnaires are useful to screen for dyscognition (fibro fog) in patients with FM, but full neuropsychological testing may be required to delineate the extent of cognitive dysfunction. The FIQR is a tool used to assess fibromyalgia intensity and track progress over time in response to treatment. It is important to notice that these assessments go well beyond rating your pain from 0 to 10.

Revised Fibromyalgia Impact Questionnaire (FIQR)

Duration of FM symptoms (years): _____

Time since FM was first diagnosed (years): _____

Directions: For each of the following 9 questions check the box from 0 to 10 that best indicates how much your fibromyalgia made it difficult to perform each of the following activities during the past 7 days. If you did not perform a particular activity in the last 7 days, rate the difficulty for the last time you performed the activity. If you can't perform an activity, check the last box.

Brush or comb your hair	No difficulty ▢▢▢▢▢▢▢▢▢▢▢ Very Difficult
Walk continuously for 20 minutes	No difficulty ▢▢▢▢▢▢▢▢▢▢▢ Very Difficult
Prepare a homemade meal	No difficulty ▢▢▢▢▢▢▢▢▢▢▢ Very Difficult
Vacuum, scrub or sweep floors	No difficulty ▢▢▢▢▢▢▢▢▢▢▢ Very Difficult

Lift and carry a bag full of groceries	No difficulty ☐☐☐☐☐☐☐☐☐☐ Very Difficult
Climb one flight of stairs	No difficulty ☐☐☐☐☐☐☐☐☐☐ Very Difficult
Change bed sheets	No difficulty ☐☐☐☐☐☐☐☐☐☐ Very Difficult
Sit in a chair for 45 minutes	No difficulty ☐☐☐☐☐☐☐☐☐☐ Very Difficult
Go shopping for groceries	No difficulty ☐☐☐☐☐☐☐☐☐☐ Very Difficult

Sub-total ___ /3= _____

Directions: For each of the following 2 questions, check the box that best describes the overall impact of your fibromyalgia over the last 7 days.

Fibromyalgia prevented me from accomplishing goals for the week	Never ☐☐☐☐☐☐☐☐☐☐ Always
I was completely overwhelmed by my fibromyalgia symptoms	Never ☐☐☐☐☐☐☐☐☐☐ Always

Sub-total: _____

pain. This analgesic effect, termed "diffuse noxious inhibitory controls" (DNIC), has been consistently observed to be attenuated or absent in groups of FM patients as compared to healthy controls. Someone unaffected by FM gradually has a diminishment of the sensation of pain throughout the body and localizes to the painful stimulus. In fibromyalgia patients, they do not turn off the diffuse pain.

The DNIC response is believed to be partly mediated by descending opiate acting pathways and, in part, descending serotonin and norepinephrine acting pathways. The biochemical and imaging findings supporting increased (or intact) activity of existing opioid acting pathways in FM are consistent with the anecdotal clinical experience that opioids are generally ineffective analgesics in patients with FM. There is also some evidence that blocking the opioid receptors with naloxone, which is used to reverse heroin overdoses, is beneficial.

In contrast, studies have shown the opposite for serotonergic and noradrenergic activity in FM. Where the overactivity of opioid activity occurs in fibromyalgia, low activity occurs in the neuro-transmitters serotonin and epinephrine. For example, the waste product of norepinephrine, 3-methoxy-4-hydroxyphenethylamine (MHPG), is lower in the spinal fluid of FM patients. Similarly, patients with FM have been shown to have reduced serum levels of serotonin and its precursor, L-tryptophan, and the principal serotonin metabolite, 5-HIAA, in the spinal fluid. Further evidence supporting deficiencies in this mechanism comes from treatment studies. Nearly any type of compound simultaneously raises both serotonin and norepinephrine (tricyclics, duloxetine, milnacipran, tramadol) and is efficacious in treating FM and related conditions.

Studies have not only demonstrated hypersensitivity to pain, but fibromyalgia patients are also hypersensitive to heat, cold, electrical shocks to the skin and muscle, reduced blood flow (ischemia), and salt injections into the muscle, among others. Further, allodynia, an increased intensity to damaging stimulation, such as warmth, cold, and pressure, has been documented. Temporal summation has been demonstrated by using heat, cold, and intramuscular electric stimuli. As often complained by FM patients, sensitivity to noise has been shown in a human pain laboratory by using a noise generator.

One of the mechanisms for central sensitization occurs through repetitive painful stimuli. This temporal summation of the second pain (TSSP) occurs in those with FM more than those without FM. TSSP was demonstrated in a study where patients were divided between those who had FM and those who did not. They each received repetitive painful heat shocks to the thumb area of the palm. The results are shown in the following illustration.

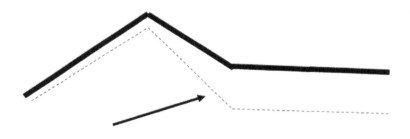

After the initial painful stimulus, pain levels in those unaffected by fibromyalgia drop, but levels persist in those with fibromyalgia.

A similar study injected saltwater into the calf muscles of those with and without FM to see if there were differences in pain responses. The results showed that after about 10 to 12 minutes, those without FM were able to filter out the pain and reported decreasing levels of pain compared to those with FM who had higher levels of pain persisting. The FM patient experiences the world more unfiltered and unbuffered.

One way to understand the temporal summation of pain is by filling two balloons with air. Both initially get inflated to the same pressure. The amount of pressure represents the experience of pain. Both balloons have holes in them through which they leak out air, but those with FM have smaller holes and do not leak air out as quickly as those without FM. Painful stimuli do not fade as quickly in those with fibromyalgia when repetitive stimuli are received. Many patients with FM may have had surgery to fix a joint problem but still have a considerable amount of pain out of proportion to what the surgeon would expect. The pain lasts much past the time most would have recovered.

"Lisa" had a traumatic injury to her ankle which didn't lead to a fracture but significant bruising to the bones and ligaments. What made it different for her was that her pain was quite disabling for several months afterwards compared to someone who did not have the tendency to FM who would have recovered in a few weeks. Her injury also took her off her exercise routine. Transitioning to alternative exercising like swimming or biking could have reduced the time to recovery. What wasn't apparent at the time was her untreated adult ADHD that likely was a barrier to her recovery. She did gradually increase her activity climbing back to her baseline activity and pain levels.

Another study compared the effect of thumbnail pressure and sound intensity between those with and without FM. It demonstrated that there was more distress at lower levels of pressure and sound levels than those without FM. These studies indicate that there is an intensified response to all kinds of stimuli and not just mechanical.

Pain is only one way those suffering experience distress. In addition to pain, other sensory systems are also heightened, including light and cold. It may be a mom who has small children enthusiastically playing, but she feels very distressed by the noise. It may be the cold of winter that is especially uncomfortable compared to a healthy person. For many with FM, the smells of everyday odors become almost intolerable. Sound and smell sensitivity are familiar to those of you who have suffered migraines. This hypersensitivity is not surprising because migraines are under the umbrella of fibromyalgia pain disorders. Light sensitivity has also been found to differ in those with FM. FM patients report discomfort at a lower threshold of around 100 LUX compared to about 1,000 LUX in those without.

Lighting condition	LUX
Pitch Black	0
Very Dark	11
Dark Indoors	51
Dim indoors	201
Normal indoors	401
Bright indoors	1,000
Cloudy outdoors	10,000
Direct Sunlight	30,000

This difference appears to occur due to modulation of light input in the brainstem. These findings are consistent with higher FIQR scores (Fibromyalgia Impact Questionnaire-Revised) for sensitivity to loud noises, bright lights, odors, or cold. Other areas of the brain are involved in modulation of pain. The area of the brain known as the insula appears to be quite involved in both sensing and responding to the sensory stimuli. Regions of the insula are proposed to be involved in an interoceptive system activated in response to sensations arising from within the body, including pain, temperature, itch, sensual touch, hunger, thirst, and muscular and visceral sensations. This interoceptive system may be involved in the sensitivity to various stimuli observed in persons with FM. Interoception is the inside awareness or sense of the internal state of the body. This can be both conscious and non-conscious. It can be thought of as, "How do I feel?"

Other research on FM includes altered levels of substance P and glutamate. Levels of substance P are higher as well as levels of glutamate, an excitatory neurotransmitter, are twice as high in those with fibromyalgia. The spinal fluid of those with FM has high levels of opioids. For opioids to work, the dopamine system has to work properly. When spinal fluid is pulled out of those with FM and examined, many endorphins (natural opiates) are detected. A study involving rats involved blocking the effect of dopamine by giving a medication. The rats were given morphine, and then were shocked. Pain levels were higher than if they weren't given the dopamine blocker. Clinically this is important because those with ADHD have naturally lower levels of dopamine activity. There are antipsychotic medications that block dopamine and could have an impact on FM symptoms.

Take home points:
- **Muscle tenderness is the hallmark of FM, but the findings in multiple studies suggest that people with FM display sensitivity to many sensory stimuli.**

- Study findings suggest that FM is associated with a global central nervous system augmentation of sensory information.
- People with FM have a vigilant, "very protective nervous system."
- FM patients experience the world less filtered.

Chapter 2
Catastrophizing

People with fibromyalgia feel as if their control of pain is much more outside of their power. They feel less ability to control their pain. In 'Sur L'eau, novelist Maupassant (1875) wrote concerning his experience with migraines, "*Migraine is an atrocious torment, one of the worst in the world, weakening the nerves, driving one mad, scattering one's thoughts to the winds and impairing the memory. So terrible are these headaches that I can do nothing but lie on the couch and try to dull the pain by sniffing ether.*" Ether was one of the earliest anesthesia medications.

Maupassant's words describe the torment of pain, emotional distress, and the disability that pain brings to his life. He feels overwhelmed by his suffering and helpless to deal with it. He surrenders to the pain and seeks chemical means of dulling it. Today's specialists on the psychology of pain would argue that Maupassant's 'catastrophic thinking' about his pain likely played a role in heightening the intensity of the pain he experienced.

Catastrophizing is defined as: "an exaggerated negative mental set brought to bear during actual or anticipated painful experience." Pain catastrophizing, or responses to pain that characterize it as awful, horrible, and unbearable, is increasingly recognized as a significant contributor to the experience of pain. Studies have found catastrophizing to be associated with illness and pain-related disability independent of the influence of depression. Studies have observed that catastrophizing alone accounted for 47% of the variance in predicting chronic pain development from an acute pain episode. Although the precise mechanisms by which catastrophizing influences the experience of pain are not clear, it is thought that this cognitive style influences the attentional focus on painful events. Persons who catastrophize have more difficulty shifting their center of attention away from uncomfortable or threatening stimuli. This interferes with their ability to stay on track for goals they have set up.

If you have FM and plan to get 5 to 6 moderately challenging projects done during the day, you are more likely to struggle with feeling overwhelmed, getting distracted, and only completing one of the goals. You are generally more likely to appraise new situations and challenges as being more threatening or harmful. This relationship between catastrophizing and pain has been shown in hundreds of studies. A significant connection between catastrophizing and pain-related outcomes has been observed in numerous pain samples. These have included patients with rheumatoid arthritis, osteoarthritis, fibromyalgia, sickle cell disease, soft tissue injuries, neuropathic pain, dental patients, and patients recovering from surgery.

The relationship between catastrophizing and pain appears to emerge early in life and has been observed in children as young as seven years. It has been observed across a wide range of clinical and experimental pain-eliciting situations and shows remarkable consistency. Implicit in this work is the view that catastrophizing is causally related to pain. The pattern of findings appears to support the causal or, at least, the antecedent status of catastrophizing.

For example, catastrophizing, assessed while individuals are in a pain-free state, predicts future pain ratings made in response to damaging tissue stimulation. Catastrophizing scores obtained one week or ten weeks before a painful procedure predicted future pain ratings. Catastrophizing prospectively predicted pain ratings in arthritis patients six months later, even when controlling for initial pain ratings.

Reductions in catastrophizing have been shown to predict decreases in pain and disability prospectively.

Since pain catastrophizing, or characterizations of pain as awful, horrible, and unbearable, is increasingly being recognized as an important factor in the experience of pain, researchers decided to look for differences in brain responses using fMRI. The purpose of this investigation was to examine the association between catastrophizing, as measured by the Coping Strategies Questionnaire Catastrophizing Subscale, and brain responses to blunt pressure assessed by functional MRI among 29 subjects with fibromyalgia. Since catastrophizing has been suggested to augment pain perception through enhanced attention to painful stimuli, and heightened emotional responses to pain, they hypothesized that catastrophizing would be positively associated with activation in structures believed to be involved in these aspects of pain processing.

Their findings suggest that pain catastrophizing, independent of the influence of depression, is significantly associated with increased activity in brain areas related to anticipation of pain (medial frontal cortex, cerebellum), attention to pain (dorsal ACC, dorsolateral prefrontal cortex), emotional aspects of pain (claustrum, closely connected to amygdala) and motor control. These results support the hypothesis that catastrophizing influences pain perception through altering attention and anticipation, while heightening emotional responses to pain. Activation associated with catastrophizing in motor areas of the brain may reflect expressive responses to pain that are associated with greater pain catastrophizing.

The Role of Attention

Attention to pain symptoms appears to be one of the ways catastrophizing contributes to increased physical and emotional distress. For example, the rumination subscale of the Pain Catastrophizing Scale is most highly correlated with pain outcomes. The endorsement of items, such as "I keep thinking about how much it hurts" and "I can't seem to keep it out of my mind," has been most consistently associated with more severe pain symptoms. For example, the rumination component of pain catastrophizing contributed significant unique variance to the prediction of pain intensity during dental hygiene treatments. Other studies reported that only the rumination added substantial prediction of pain-related disability in a sample of patients with soft tissue injuries.

Several investigators have discussed the importance of attentional mechanisms associated with pain catastrophizing. Pain catastrophizers showed more significant interference on attention-demanding tasks than non-pain-catastrophizers in anticipation of a pain stimulus onset. Another study showed that pain catastrophizers were unsuccessful in using cognitive attention diversion coping strategies to reduce pain. Similarly, another study suggested that pain catastrophizers have more difficulty diverting attention away from pain. Another study indicated that excessive focus on pain sensations may lead to the facilitation of pain access into consciousness and the magnification of painful feelings. Neuroimaging studies have shown that brain areas responsible for attentional modulation are more likely to be activated in high catastrophizers during the experience of pain.

As I will discuss in more detail later, these are likely explained by higher rates of ADHD in those with fibromyalgia-like pain conditions. Findings suggest that pain catastrophizing may facilitate processes involved in temporal summation. Other studies have also established a link between pain catastrophizing and the operation of endogenous pain-modulatory systems. This association between pain catastrophizing and diffuse noxious inhibitory controls, a psychophysical measure of endogenous pain inhibition, was demonstrated. Activation associated with catastrophizing in motor areas of the brain may reflect emotional reactions to pain that are associated with more considerable pain catastrophizing.

Part of catastrophizing is the sense of feeling overwhelmed and unable to sort out a plan to get through the difficulty. Most of my patients with coexisting ADHD and fibromyalgia show high levels of feeling overwhelmed when they are untreated compared to low levels when their ADHD is treated.

On a scale of 0 to 10, with 0 being not at all and 10 being very high, how overwhelmed on average do you feel?

If you have FM that is not under control or ADHD, you are likely to report levels of 7 to 10. It is not uncommon for some to report a level of 12/10. Treatment of ADHD with psychostimulants will reduce the sense of feeling overwhelmed for most of those with ADHD. If they also have FM, then the FIQR score also typically drops. Attention to pain and difficulty attending to other tasks are consistent with the higher rates of ADHD in fibromyalgia-like pain conditions.

Chapter 3
Diagnosis of Fibromyalgia

The diagnosis, like all medical diagnoses, starts with a meticulous history. Ninety percent of all diagnoses are made by history, with about 9% through an additional physical exam and the remainder through lab and imaging testing. The 2016 fibromyalgia criteria as noted in this chapter are used to help make the diagnosis. The symptoms and intensity of fibromyalgia typically vary over time. For example, during the summer months in Wisconsin, the levels may be lower compared to elevated fibromyalgia symptoms during the winter. Levels can even vary from day to day and week to week. This variability is important to keep in mind when making a diagnosis.

FM is similar to most syndromes or disorders that use criteria as guides to complement a thorough history and physical exam. An astute clinician uses tests to confirm their suspicions, make sure they aren't missing a rare disorder, or alter the treatment plan. For example, someone may have severe episodic headaches preceded by distorted vision, fatigue progressing to a crescendoing, pulsating headache with light and sound sensitivity, and a plateau of moderate to severe pain that lasts from a few hours to 3 days. She describes feeling fine in-between episodes. On a careful exam, she has a normal general and neurologic exam.

Although an MRI could be done, it wouldn't be necessary to make the diagnosis of migraines. A structural MRI would show a healthy brain, but that doesn't dismiss that she indeed has real suffering and is making up all the symptoms. We learned earlier about the abnormal findings found in research settings using functional MRI tracking the blood flow in the brain of those with chronic fibromyalgia-like pain disorders compared to those who don't.

Another example of widespread pain and fatigue may be seen in patients presenting with a viral syndrome or acute hepatitis. However, compared to fibromyalgia-like syndromes, these symptoms typically do not last for more than three months. Recently being in a car crash with multiple diffuse injuries also would not qualify for fibromyalgia. A thorough history and physical examination are usually sufficient to distinguish fibromyalgia from other conditions in the differential diagnosis. The only abnormal finding on exam may be tender points or some distress to a brightly lit exam room. Some blood tests such as a thyroid level, sedimentation rate, or CBC, sometimes are ordered to rule out other problems like hypothyroidism, polymyalgia rheumatica, or anemia.

2016 Fibromyalgia Diagnostic Criteria

1. Widespread pain index (WPI) and symptom severity score (SSS) WPI≥7andSSS≥5OR WPI4-6andSSS≥9
2. Generalized pain: pain in 4/5 regions
3. Symptoms present ≥ 3 months

The fibromyalgia diagnosis can now be made irrespective of other diagnoses (you do not need to rule out all other conditions that could explain the symptoms, if criteria 1-3 are all met).

Widespread pain index (WPI)

In the past week, where have you had pain?
(check all that apply)

Left upper region	Right upper region
Left jaw	Right jaw
Left shoulder	Left shoulder
Left upper arm	Left upper arm
Left lower arm	Left lower arm

Left lower region	Right lower region
Left hip or buttock	Right hip or buttock
Left upper leg	Right upper leg
Left lower leg	Right lower leg

Axial Region
Neck
Upper back
Lower back
Chest
Abdomen

Total: _____ WPI score (add up boxes checked, 0 to 19)

Symptoms Severity Score (SSS)

For each of the following, for the past week, rate each symptom.

	0=No problem	1=slight or mild problem	2+moderate, considerable often present	3=severe, pervasive, continuous, life disturbing
Fatigue				
Waking unrefreshed				
Cognitive symptoms				

Cognitive difficulties include trouble concentrating, forgetfulness, and disorganized or slow thinking.

In the past week, have you been bothered by any of the following?

	0= No problem	1= problem
Headaches		
Pain or cramps in the lower abdomen		
Depression		

Total SSS: _____ (0 to 12)

Summary:

1. **Criterion 1 is met if you have EITHER** or WPI ≥ 7 and SSS ≥ 5 or **WPI 4-6 and SSS ≥ 9.**
2. **Generalized pain met if you checked pain in 4/5 regions (not including items in italics)**
3. **Symptoms present ≥ 3 months**

Fibromyalgia is diagnosed if you meet all 3 criteria 1-3, independent of whether other diagnoses contribute to these symptoms. This is new: FMS diagnosis used to require that there be no other diagnosis to explain the findings.

This new diagnostic proposal is based on the conceptualization of FM as a dimensional syndrome which includes five dimensions:

1. Core Diagnostic Criteria, defined as the presence of pain in six or more body sites from a total of nine possible localizations, sleep disturbance, and fatigue
2. Common Features, like tenderness, dyscognition (e.g., trouble concentrating, forgetfulness, and disorganized or slow thinking), musculoskeletal stiffness, and environmental sensitivity or hyper-vigilance
3. Common Medical and Psychiatric Comorbidities like chronic fatigue syndrome, irritable bowel syndrome, chronic pelvic pain, interstitial cystitis, orofacial conditions, chronic headaches, depression, anxiety disorders, central sleep apnea, restless leg syndrome, etc.
4. Neurobiological, Psychosocial and Functional Consequences, which includes general outcome, functional disability, social and medical cost of FMS, morbidity, and mortality; and
5. Putative Neurobiological and Psychosocial Mechanisms, Risk Factors, and Protective Factors that focus on risk factors, comorbidities, and pathophysiology aspects.

It can sometimes be a challenge diagnosing FM, and often there is a long delay of years and multiple doctor visits, to multiple doctors, before the diagnosis is made. The primary care physician should establish a diagnosis of FM as early as possible, without need for confirmation by a specialist, and communicate this diagnosis to the patient. Repeated investigations after diagnosis should be avoided unless driven by the onset of new symptoms or signs on physical examination. This continued testing can augment anxiety and lead to frustration and distrust of the medical system's ability to care for and treat them. It also can lead to mounting medical bills through unnecessary tests and procedures.

We rely on tests to see if someone has an illness like rheumatoid arthritis. However, sometimes testing can lead to unintended consequences. For example, an imaging study reveals incidental and tangential findings that are not likely causing the symptoms. Physicians may make an error known as an anchoring error or bias where an initial diagnosis ends the pursuit of other possible causes. Someone may have been seen for chronic neck or back pain, with an MRI showing a bulge or arthritis in the spine. With disk disease or arthritis given as the cause of their problems, multiple treatments, including injections and surgery, may be attempted with little or no improvement.

This diagnostic error concludes that the bulge is causing pain and underappreciating the effect of an augmented pain modulation in those with FM and related syndromes. Most people who have bulging discs or herniations don't even have pain. This can lead to years of unnecessary suffering and incorrect treatment. It is like the police arresting an innocent bystander who is sentenced to prison for a crime they didn't commit—meanwhile, the atrocities continue, and the real criminal is roaming free.

Key point: The 2016 fibromyalgia criteria as noted in this chapter are used to help make the diagnosis. This is similar to many disorders that are used as a guide in addition to a thorough history and physical exam.

How common is fibromyalgia-like pain?

Fibromyalgia is suffered by about 3 to 6% of the world's population. However, central/fibromyalgia-like pain is much more common, and to some extent, occurs in up to fifty percent of people. For some, it is very mild, such as the occasional tension headache. Others are at the complete other ends of the spectrum with debilitating pain making it tough to function. Fibromyalgia prevalence estimates can vary fourfold depending on the diagnostic criteria applied.

Fibromyalgia pain is also on a spectrum from clearly meeting all the criteria to meeting many but not most. In an extensive study of chronic pain, the prevalence was quite high, derived from 7 studies, ranging from 35% to 51%. The number of people with moderate to severely disabling chronic pain based on four studies, ranging from 10% to 14%. Twelve studies divided chronic pain prevalence by age group, demonstrating a trend towards increasing levels with advancing age from 14% in 18- to 25-year-olds to 62% in the over 75 age group.

However, the prevalence of chronic pain in young people (18 to 39 years old) may be as high as 30%. Women are more often diagnosed, probably because they are more likely to seek medical care. The ratio is likely close to 2:1 of women to men who have fibromyalgia. The amount of chronic pain probably goes up with age because of overall decreased exercise due to a variety of factors. There may be less time as work and family responsibilities vie for attention. Accrual of injuries or joint problems from wear and tear over time, without being aware of the need for regular exercise to buffer their chronic pain. Accumulated injuries and higher levels of stress over time likely account for increased levels of chronic pain over time as well.

Genetics

Fibromyalgia-type pain commonly occurs in families. Fibromyalgia-type pain are those pain disorders that include pain amplification and central nervous system sensitization features. This will be discussed more thoroughly in the chapter on the "faces of fibromyalgia." Typically, one suffering from fibromyalgia type pain has a family member with the diagnosis or at least symptoms of one of the chronic pain problems at some point in their life. There is an estimated 50% environmental component to developing centralized pain and a 50% genetic component. First degree relatives (parent or sibling) are at eight times greater risk of developing widespread pain compared to the average population.

Many may not have been clearly labeled as fibromyalgia or formally diagnosed with irritable bowel, migraines, or tension headaches but have had symptoms consistent with those problems. They may have had a chronically "sensitive stomach," but never told it was irritable bowel syndrome or dyspepsia or had self-diagnosed lactose intolerance. There may have been relatives with a history of chronic back, knee, or neck pain. Your father may have had migraines, but now you have irritable bowel syndrome. The common thread tying them together is inheriting a more sensitive nervous system.

ADHD appears to play a big role and also is strongly genetic with an autosomal dominant pattern. This means that if a parent has ADHD, half of his or her children would likely develop ADHD. The symptoms of fibromyalgia can fluctuate over time in an individual. There are some common themes we will talk more about later. One pattern is that the overall pain and life disruption is the lowest when you have been the most consistently active, under the least amount of stress, eating higher levels of whole-foods plant-based foods, and have been sleeping the best.

We will read more later about the causes, other coexisting illnesses, and the treatments available. Fibromyalgia often coexists with other chronic, painful conditions generally classified as functional somatic syndromes. These include migraine or tension headaches, irritable bowel syndrome, chronic fatigue syndrome, interstitial cystitis (painful bladder syndrome), chronic pelvic pain, cyclical vomiting syndrome,

POTS, ADHD, and temporomandibular joint disorder among many others.

These disorders are more prevalent in patients with fibromyalgia but are also believed to have common central nervous system mechanisms and tend to cluster in affected patients. The recognition and management of these comorbid disorders can help in achieving treatment goals. Regular physical activity, weight loss, and treatment of mood and sleep disturbances may be protective against fibromyalgia and other chronic pain conditions.

A study looking at twins with chronic pain syndromes, including widespread chronic pain, irritable bowel syndrome, chronic pelvic pain, and spinal pain, shared an inheritability of 66%. Genes shape our neural structures, immunological and endocrinological processes, and, subsequently, our behavior and experiences. However, this is not just a one-way effect; the environment can also impact our genes and alter gene expression known as epigenetics. There is increasing evidence that social experiences and contextual factors (e.g., stress and abuse) can have long-lasting effects by impacting gene expression and consequently manifesting behavioral changes.

Genes are involved in the production of serotonin such as tryptophan hydroxylase and β2-adrenoceptor gene (ADRB2), which affects nerve signaling through adrenaline type signals. Other genes involved include control of enzymes such as COMT Catechol-O-methyltransferase, one of several enzymes that degrade adrenaline-type signaling chemicals known as catecholamines (dopamine, epinephrine, and norepinephrine), catechol estrogens, and various drugs and substances having a similar underlying structure.

Other environmental factors that play a significant role include diet choices. Studies and anecdotal reports show that a diet high in whole plant-based foods can lessen symptoms. Exercise also plays a considerable role. People with FM fare better with consistently higher levels of regular exercise than those without FM. Stay tuned for more further discussion in section 2 on treatment and management of FM.

Take home message:
- **Genes can have a powerful impact by affecting levels of neurotransmitters involved in pain regulation.**
- **The environment affects the expression of genes known as epigenetics.**

Have you ever heard someone say, "I carry my stress in my _____" and the blank is for some location in their body?

In one sense, this is what is meant by central pain sensitization or fibromyalgia type pain. For many people, this may be a dull tension headache. I often hear a story from my patients where they report that when they're not "taking care of themselves," they get neck pain or back pain. What do they mean by not "taking care of themselves"? That usually means that when they're under a fair amount of stress, they aren't sleeping well, exercising regularly, and eating well. They can sense their body doesn't feel right. They report increased pain and soreness. People can have chest, arm, or neck soreness. "Is this my heart or fibromyalgia type pain?" Usually, fibromyalgia pain is worse at rest, and the longer someone is resting. If you get up and go for a walk or other exercise, the pain will diminish and possibly even go away **while** being active.

In contrast, pain caused by blockages in the heart will intensify as the activity level increases. If your chest pain would get worse with exercise, make sure you see your doctor, but if it gets better, then this reinforces that you likely have more fibromyalgia type pain. For most people with FM, the pain seems to get worse after they are done exercising. Many people may report, "sometimes, if I am distracted or busy doing things, I don't notice the pain as much." For many, the pain will be worse after they exercise, especially if the exercise has been more intense and more prolonged than they are accustomed. It is crucial to discriminate that the pain didn't get worse while you were exercising and you felt better, versus increased pain after you stopped exercising.

"John" saw me twice for atypical chest pain. Atypical chest pain is a term used medically to describe chest pain that does not meet the classic symptoms of a blocked artery to the heart known as angina. Atypical chest pain also doesn't have other causes such as pneumonia or a clear injury to the muscles or ribs. I had seen him 6 months previously for atypical chest pain and gave him reassurance that he was fine. Often that is all that is needed as the pain is often self-limited and goes away within a few weeks. He was 24 years old and had a sedentary job working as a computer programmer.

He now returned again 6 months later with persistent symptoms. He did report physical activity lessened his symptoms. He was working at home during the COVID pandemic allowing him to have more time to exercise as he had been spending about an hour commuting previously. He was able to take 30 to 45-minute walks over lunch and had noticed he felt better. His blood pressure and cholesterol were at very low risk levels. He didn't smoke. He had no injury, and his exam was normal except for some tender points in the upper outer chest regions, mid-trapezius regions, along his paraspinal and anterior neck muscles. This was beginning to look more like fibromyalgia-like pain.

I inquired about his sleep which he reported as chronically poor. He had a hard time falling asleep due to uncomfortable feelings in his legs that were hard to describe. The symptoms worsened the longer he was in bed, and he tossed and turned throughout the night. He momentarily felt better when he moved or got out of bed and walked around only for it to return when he laid back down. He had these symptoms going back to early childhood. His mother and sister, "Cassie" had similar symptoms but never diagnosed with RLS which is all too common. His maternal grandfather also had RLS symptoms that were never identified or treated. John also felt tired during the day.

He was started on gabapentin and was able to fall asleep, stay asleep, and wake up refreshed in the morning. The chest pain also went away. He felt more energy and was exercising more. He also started eating more of a whole-foods plant-based diet which helped his stomach feel less bloated.

He shared this new revelation with his mother and Cassie. They had read the handout on restless leg syndrome and felt the symptoms of RLS resonated with what she was struggling with as well.

Cassie also had struggled with painful menstrual periods, leg pains and some headaches. She ran track which seemed to lessen her symptoms. She wanted to get an appointment before college, but I was booked out. Not wanting to delay her suffering I saw her 2 weeks later. She had the same symptoms. For as long as Cassie could remember, she could never sleep well. Before age 5 her mom reported Cassie had difficulty falling and staying asleep and that her legs were bothering her. Mom told her she had growing pains. I checked to make sure she didn't have iron deficiency that sometimes can cause restless leg syndrome.

Typically, strong familial cases are due to an inherited deficiency of dopamine levels in parts of the brain that affect leg movements and sleep. She had been to her pediatrician in the past for leg pains and painful menstrual cramps but the connection to underlying restless leg syndrome was never made. She started on gabapentin and had the same response as her brother John. She no longer had uncomfortable sensations in her legs with the urge to move and restless unrefreshing sleep.

The Purpose of pain

A question to ask is, why do we have pain in the first place? Functionally, pain is designed to be an alarm system alerting us to something that is injuring our body. Unfortunately, with fibromyalgia, the alarm has become very sensitive and triggered at lower thresholds. The sensitivity is affected by several factors, including sleep, stress, activity, hormone levels, genetics, and diet.

Many have experienced physical trauma in the form of a car accident. They were doing well until suddenly and dramatically; they developed pain activating the acute pain due to bone and muscle trauma, but after the injuries have healed, the chronic pain circuits remain turned on. During the recovery, the body rests to recover, which is useful if you sprained an ankle or developed Achilles tendonitis. Still, for those with chronic fibromyalgia, the reduced activity leads to a downward spiral. The exercise which helped suppress the pain sensitivity is no longer active.

Let's look at how this reduction in activity dramatically played out with "Linda."

"Linda" had been working in an active, hands-on factory job and exercised 90 minutes a day after work until she was stung by a bee leading to anaphylaxis. She needed to be intubated and placed on a ventilator for five days. After "Linda" recovered, she found herself in a state of profound fatigue and muscle pain. Her anaphylaxis had been completely healed, but she was suffering in other ways.

What had happened? How did a perfectly healthy person develop severe symptoms in less than a week?

In a way, she treated her predisposition to fibromyalgia without even knowing it by having an active job and active free time that, when taken away, unleashed her genetic susceptibility to fibromyalgia. She went through months of diffuse pain and was not working or exercising, further prolonging her recovery. By the time I saw her, she had months of frustration despite seeing multiple doctors. I took a careful history and thorough assessment. I did the Fibromyalgia impact score (FIQR), which revealed she was in the severe range. She had a hard time just getting things done around the house. She felt a mental fog and was very unmotivated. Her energy was low, especially compared to the very active lifestyle she had been in before the bee sting. Her irritable bowel syndrome was also acting up. Her migraines and tension headaches were frequent as well. She struggled just to get the essentials done of caring for her family at home, which was becoming more and more difficult.

Because about 50% of people with FM have ADHD, which is even higher in those with elevated levels of functional impairment when measured through the FIQR, I evaluated her for ADHD. She had a history of academic struggles going back to grade school with difficulty focusing and staying on cognitively challenging tasks with easy distraction that continued through high school. The WHO (World Health Organization) adult ADHD questionnaire supported the diagnosis of ADHD.

Also, she reported insomnia with uncomfortable feelings in her legs that worsened the longer she laid in bed. They were accompanied by an irresistible urge to move the legs, which helped temporarily alleviate her symptoms. She frequently woke through the night, tossing and turning a lot. She had a history of "growing pains" at night as a child. I diagnosed her with RLS. As severely affected as she was, she needed more than just a pep talk and encouragement to relax more, meditate, and just get out there and be more active. She needed treatment to get out of the deep hole she had collapsed into.

Appropriate medications targeting these underlying untreated problems were required to help her get on her feet. I felt that if we could bridge her with medications and then through a gradual return to her before high levels of activity, she could get back to functioning as well and even better than before.

Her restless leg was treated with gabapentin at night, which helped her feel more rested in the AM, but she still hurt during the day. Duloxetine, which increases the serotonin and norepinephrine levels, gradually put her on the road to recovery.

For some with FM syndromes, they too may have compensated well initially but had a gradual worsening of their symptoms over time. It may have started with being less active during pregnancy and disrupted sleep with caring for a newborn. Many don't achieve the same level of exercise they had before pregnancy due to time constraints and the fatigue associated with their fibromyalgia symptoms. Symptoms of anxiety and depression often occur with time as frustration builds.

Linda's pain levels improved, but she still had a lot of fatigue, mental fog, and low motivation. She was started on a form of long-acting methylphenidate for her ADHD, and the dose was adjusted. She reported a significant increase in her ability to get things done, which I like to call TCB, taking care of business. She didn't have a sense of euphoria or a high but was able to get things done. She was motivated. The more she was able to accomplish, the more her self-confidence and optimism grew. She catastrophized less. An evening dose was added as she struggled more in the evening to complete projects and with pain. This addition improved her functioning.

What happened to her activity level? Without having to put her on a specific exercise regimen, she was already more active just by doing housework. Her activity counter showed that she went from about 1000 steps a day to approximately 4000-7000 steps a day. Her FIQR level had now dropped into a low range from the high levels before *treatment. She no longer felt overwhelmed and was on the path to not just surviving with fibromyalgia but thriving with fibromyalgia.*

She had gotten the proverbial monkeys off her back, which were untreated RLS, ADHD, and had medication to boost her genetically lower levels of serotonin and norepinephrine. They all worked in concert to lift her out of the quicksand encasing her onto solid ground with better functioning and less pain. She was then able to consistently exercise, complete tasks, and feel better.

"Fibro fog"

"Fibro fog" for many is more frustrating than the pain they experience with FM. "Fibro fog" refers to the symptoms of short-term memory loss, misplacing objects, becoming easily distracted from goals by irrelevant distractions, forgetting plans, difficulty carrying on conversations, and difficulty remembering new information. These symptoms overlap with those of ADHD.

This overlap is more than a coincidence. Studies have shown what I have observed in many of my patients with FM, where nearly half of those with fibromyalgia tested positive for ADHD based on the WHO organization adult ADHD screening. This questionnaire can underestimate when used alone, so a careful history of teasing out nuances is essential. It is estimated that 90% of adults with ADHD have not been diagnosed or are not being treated. One of the symptoms many with ADHD have is a sense of being overwhelmed, which can heighten their pain. They have difficulty distracting themselves from the pain by maintaining their attention on different things. This observation helps explain why they experience pain at higher levels.

The study also showed that those with the highest FIQR scores (Fibromyalgia Impact Questionnaire Revised) were ten times more likely to have ADHD than those with the lowest scores. This finding is consistent with the observation that those with fibromyalgia need to be more active than the average person to have normal levels of pain. We will talk more about fibro fog and fatigue when discussing chronic fatigue syndrome later in the book. There also will be an upcoming chapter diving deeper into ADHD, Attention Deficit Hyperactivity Disorder.

Chapter 4
Stress

When patients were surveyed on the likely cause(s) of their fibromyalgia, four themes were generated:

1.   Bodily assault, ill-health, and life change
2.   Emotional trauma and distress
3.   Stress and vulnerability
4.   Explaining and authenticating fibromyalgia.

What's clear from many patients suffering from FM is that stress plays a significant role. You have read about underlying mechanisms that play a role in FM, but how does stress influence your reality? Let's dig deeper and see how these dots are connected.

An online survey asked those with fibromyalgia what caused their condition. Commonly cited were car accidents, skeletal injuries, and nerve problems, with many participants highlighting the importance of damage to the cervical spine. Bodily assaults included accidents, third-person attacks, surgery, infections, poisons, and allergens. Isolated incidents were described, but accounts more often suggested cumulative physical events:

"I have had multiple bodily ailments – Bus crash, a back injury in a fall, heavy lifting during employment, physical assault – which I feel led to my issues," said Anne, 55.

What is the role of these in fibromyalgia? Anne and others like her had significant events. They recall the development and crescendoing of fibromyalgia symptoms. How do these events fit in with our understanding of FM?

Let's look at the role accidents can play. These events can significantly increase fibromyalgia symptoms. There is increased pain from the injury, which is often amplified in someone with an FM patient. The protective buffer of exercise is often reduced to a dramatic level compared to their pre-accident level. Sleep may be worsened because of difficulty recovering from the accident. There may be increased anxiety and sometimes PTSD from having trouble blocking out the traumatic events.

Some of the perceived causes cited in the survey were linked to physical events, which represented significant changes in the body and life stage. Pregnancy, childbirth, hysterectomy, or menopause were frequently identified as onset events.

"The extreme tiredness, brain fog, and pain started after a planned C-section," said Kaye, a 32-year-old female. Childbirth represents a significant change that can be a blessing and a challenge in those more vulnerable to FM. Before the delivery, she may have been able to exercise at a high level and had a good sleep schedule. Time crunches, parenting, and work responsibilities, either in or out of the home, all vying for the limited time, contribute to higher FM symptoms. These restrictions are often the first time in her life that she ever had these disruptions that persisted more than a month. This change can lead to a rapid downward spiral. Poor sleep leads to worsening fatigue, which leads to less exercise, and the cycle repeats. Resilience gets tested, and often the dam breaks. If unaware of the FM, let alone how to manage it, they begin to feel overwhelmed. If they are one with untreated ADHD or RLS, it is even more challenging.

Emotional trauma and distress

"I was sexually abused as a child, my dad and husband were both alcoholics and violent, so many years of stress, pain, anger,

experiences. Another example of stress is living with someone who is consistently very harsh and unloving with their words.

Being in a high-stress work environment can also be a significant factor. I had a recent patient, *"Rebecca," who had a score of 92/100 on the fibromyalgia impact score revised (FIQR), which dropped into the 20s after quitting her job and finding a job that was lower stress. A score of 20s is mild, 40s-50s is moderate, greater than 60 is severe, and greater than 80 is extreme where people are typically on disability or unable to work. She was already on medications to help, but the only thing that changed was her work environment.* Her story demonstrates the significant effect of stress on fibromyalgia.

Other causes of stress include infection, especially a more severe infection beyond a typical common cold. One that may cause significant lethargy, fatigue, fevers, often being bed-bound, or markedly reduced activity from baseline is more likely to account for worsening struggles.

Emotional stress/distress also influences pain modulation, but like stressors in general, psychological influences on FM pain processing are quite varied. Several studies suggest that personally relevant stressors play a more salient role in symptom exacerbation in FM than more global stressors. For example, at the time of the 9/11 terrorist attacks, two studies examining daily diary monitoring in FM patients were conducted in both New York and Washington, DC. Those not personally affected by the 9/11 terrorist attack did not show an increase in FM symptoms. This means that if you were not closely affected by one who had died you didn't suffer as much as if you knew someone personally. General stress tends to be less of a problem than stress that affects you personally.

We can anticipate that living through the COVID pandemic for those with fibromyalgia may also vary depending on how it impacts the individual. If there is a job loss or increased interpersonal stress from being around an abusive spouse, pain levels can increase, whereas living closer to a supportive spouse and maintaining your job and financial security would buoy the pain. If you are/were working from home and have younger school aged children, the stress could be very high. If one or more of them has untreated ADHD which is likely as ADHD is so prevalent in those with fibromyalgia, the stress level could be very high. You may have been pulled in so many directions trying to give them academic assistance while managing your work life. Isolation also is likely to contribute to stress.

Psychological factors, such as mood and emotional state, also alter pain perception. Positive emotion, induced by humor, pleasant music, pictures, or films, reduce pain sensitivity, probably by inducing positive thoughts such that the pain stimulus is valued less threatening. Conversely, a more depressed mood may increase the subjective pain experience because individuals evaluate painful stimuli as more harmful or because no effective coping strategy is available.

In the case of FM, the biomedical status has been uniquely characterized by lower levels of positive affect, especially during stressful events. This relative absence of positive emotional resources hinders FM patients from mobilizing sufficient positive affective resources to neutralize the experience of pain and the associated negative affect. In other words, your mood is so down you have lost hope to even try to get better. I see what you mean now. Stress-related loss of positive affect might be responsible for the slow recovery from stressful events, increased stress-related fatigue, and central sensitization as a common feature of FM.

Anxiety and fear have become the primary domain of research illustrated by the statement that fear of pain may be more disabling than pain itself. This opinion documents that disability in chronic pain patients is not merely the consequence of the pain magnitude. Because the correlation of pain intensity and disability is generally low, other variables such as pain-related fear, negative affect, and catastrophizing have been implicated. Wolfe et al. [1990] examined the incidence of anxiety among FM patients in a multicenter study compared to a mixed chronic pain control group. The authors found that 45% of FM patients complained of anxiety, whereas only 21% of the chronic pain controls complained of anxiety. These results underpin the importance of anxiety.

Fear of pain that causes overestimation of pain intensity might lead to exercise avoidance. This pattern is known as a maladaptive response, AKA, a bad habit. This bad habit can lead to negative consequences like further weakening of the musculoskeletal system, disability in daily life, social isolation, and depression. Thus, chronic pain patients could be caught in a downward spiral of growing avoidance, disability, and pain. Also, pain-related fear will induce misinterpretations of any bodily sensations in a catastrophic manner (pain means danger), thus increasing pain-related anxiety.

Why is pain more threatening in FM than in other chronic pain states? FM patients consider the origin of their disease as more mysterious than low back pain patients, leading them to worry and to catastrophize their pain problems. Additionally, widespread pain of FM may interfere with daily life.

Underlying ADHD may aggravate the heightened anxiety. There also are higher rates of poorer performance at work and at home. If someone with FM also has ADHD, they are likely to have higher levels of anxiety that can serve as a positive by pushing them to accomplish what is needed but, at the same time, heightens the sensitivity to pain.

As much as being exposed to stress is exasperating, a healthy support system with family can be valuable. A study by Pedro Montoya used fibromyalgia patients, and fMRI evaluated the effect of a significant other on pain perception. When the significant other was present, FM patients reported less pain and thermal pain sensitivity. They showed diminished brain activity elicited upon tactile stimulation of a tender point compared with these levels when the patients were alone. These findings are consistent with the hypothesis that social support through the presence of a significant other can influence pain processing at the emotional, behavioral, and central nervous system levels.

In contrast, some people can feel increased pain with specific individuals. This person could be someone's spouse, parent, child, or boss, with whom they have had stressful interactions in the past.

"Randall" was referred to me by his future father-in-law. He had been struggling with mysterious unresolved severe pain. He also had been suffering from painful, frequent urination. He had severe migraine headaches three times a week, insomnia, severe diffuse body pain, and abdominal pain. He had sought help from 2 different urologists but had normal urinary tests and labs and did not improve with two empiric treatments for urinary tract infections. Empiric treatments are those that are for diseases that can't be confirmed by a test, which in Randall's case would have been a normal urinalysis and urine culture.

He had been to the Emergency Department with pain so severe they decided to get a CT scan to make sure he didn't have appendicitis, inflammatory bowel disease, cancer, or a bowel perforation or obstruction. These, along with labs and visits to his primary care doctor prior, led to no answers. When I saw him and reviewed his story, lab reports, CT results and examined him, he looked very uncomfortable lying in the dark exam room as the light had been bothering him so much. He was the picture of pain.

On exam, he was very tender with all the typical fibromyalgia tender points and had diffuse abdominal tenderness. The tenderness made me understand how the emergency room doctors were worried he had possible appendicitis or inflammatory bowel disease or infection. Through taking a comprehensive review of systems (medical checklist of symptoms), it was discovered that he had classic restless leg syndrome. He also had a history of academic struggles. The WHO adult ADHD questionnaire was used and was supportive of the diagnosis of ADHD as well.

I took the time to explain what he was experiencing and how I could help, but it wasn't going to go away immediately. He had his RLS treated with gabapentin and was started on duloxetine. His pain levels improved to a moderate level. His legs no longer bothered him and prevented him from sleeping. He still struggled with focusing on running the small family business his father had been transitioning for him to take over.

Over time, however, he continued to have stress at his position running the small family business. He was getting married soon and didn't want to bring this stress into his marriage. It was difficult working with his father. His dad was inconsistent with how he interacted with Randy. He would get frequently angry and upset. His dad also had much anxiety.

Randy's anxiety escalated to the point where he needed intensive outpatient therapy. After a week of counseling, his therapist told him that counseling was not going to help because the stressful position he had running the family's small business was the "thorn that had to be removed for him to get better." The stress was related to his father's demanding, harsh, unpredictable, and highly anxious demeanor. I asked him what it was like when his dad would walk into the office. He said he could just feel his whole-body tense up. His neck and stomach would tighten, and he felt anxiety to his core.

Randy resigned from his position running the family business and decided to work for a national delivery company as a courier. This position was much less stressful compared to the sedentary job he had running the family business. This job was very active, allowing him to get in and out of his delivery truck multiple times a day, easily achieving 10,000 steps a day. It was the perfect job for someone like Randall struggling with fibromyalgia. He also had a very supportive wife and strong religious beliefs that helped keep his mooring and see him through this as well.

After 3 1/2 years, I met Randy and his FIQR score had dropped to 16, well in the normal range. He was taking duloxetine and using gabapentin to treat his restless leg. He no longer was using the Adderall to treat his ADHD, as his new position was able to be managed without it. He thought he might need to restart if he got promoted to a supervisor position down the road. He had come a long way from the patient I had seen 3 1/2 years earlier, bound by debilitating, tortuous, unrelenting fibromyalgia, irritable bowel, bladder syndromes, and migraine headaches.

I had mentioned to Randy how ADHD, RLS, and fibromyalgia run in the family, and if he thought that his dad might also have those. He said that his dad most definitely had them both. Two people living or working together and struggling with undiagnosed and untreated fibromyalgia and ADHD isn't an uncommon scenario and is like a powder keg ready to explode. Each impulsive and then regretted harsh word, yelling, and lashing out, was fanning the fibromyalgia flames in Randy. It made me wonder what might have happened had his dad been diagnosed with fibromyalgia, RLS, and ADHD earlier in his life. Could Randy's years of frustration and pain have been avoided? How might his dad's life be different if treated years ago and now?

Other examples of stressful relationships include that of a parent and their child — both with FM and ADHD - butting heads, leading to raised voices. Therapy has limited benefits if they have a hard time thinking before they react to each other harshly. In a marriage, this can also be a problem. It is not uncommon for two spontaneous adventure-seeking couples to get married but later struggle. The spontaneity was part of the impulsive side of ADHD, and the adrenaline-seeking adventures a part of the hyperactive component.

When the mundane routine of married and working life occurs that demands longer sustained ways of coping, it can lead to frustration in one spouse towards the other. The spouse that can't be as physically active as he used to becomes more anxious. This anxiety is felt by the other spouse, which can amp up her anxiety leading to more considerable pain and unease.

Take-home points
- **Stress can have a strong impact on FM symptoms.**
- **The pain level in patients with FM can increase around certain people. This increase can be seen especially in those whose family member or work associate also has untreated FM, ADHD, or other mental health issues.**
- **No one says, "I am glad I waited years to finally get my fibromyalgia and related issues like RLS and ADHD diagnosed and treated." Instead, they wish it was dealt with earlier in life.**

Post-traumatic Stress Disorder

To date, it's thought that trauma and major life stressful events are not likely to cause FM itself but, in genetically susceptible people may increase the risk of development. Also, early life events, besides acute or prolonged traumatic stress in adulthood, may affect the brain's modulatory circuitries of pain and emotions responsible for the enhanced pain responses and co-occurring symptoms reported by patients with FM. Approximately 50% of patients with fibromyalgia also have PTSD.

Post-traumatic stress disorder (PTSD, DSM-5) is a frequent, chronic psychiatric condition whose onset typically occurs after exposure to a traumatic event, characterized by a specific set of symptoms including re-experiencing, avoidance, numbing, and arousal. Fibromyalgia patients with PTSD reported the following traumas: (64%) the death of a close friend or a family member, (9.1%) the separation from a dear friend, sentimental or family partners; (9.1%) the experience of being neglected or abandoned, having received physical or sexual abuse; (9.1%) reported to have been seriously threatened in their well-being, employment, professional, social status or economic security.

Many with FM and PTSD develop bad habits that worsen functioning. Many give up caring for themselves and staying connected with therapy and doctors. There are also higher rates of self-harm that occur. Soldiers with PTSD were 3.5 times more likely to report clinically significant levels of ADHD symptoms compared to male veterans without PTSD. If an individual has PTSD, then a physician should assess for possible coexisting ADHD.

That prompts the question, what happens if someone with PTSD and ADHD is treated with a stimulant? That was put to the test with a study looking at methylphenidate, galantamine (a medicine used to help memory in dementia patients) vs. a placebo. The results were impressive. The PTSD checklist, which assesses PTSD symptom severity, showed an average 13-point drop from a baseline level of 47. These results are more significant than what is seen in treatment with SSRIs (selective serotonin reuptake inhibitors, commonly used to treat anxiety and depression disorders.)

The checklist questions rate how much they have been bothered from not at all, a 1, to 5 for extremely bothered.

- Repeated, disturbing memories, thoughts, or images of a stressful experience from the past?
- Suddenly acting or feeling as if a stressful experience were happening again (as if you were reliving it)?
- Feeling very upset when something reminded you of a stressful experience from the past?
- Having physical reactions (e.g., heart pounding, trouble breathing or sweating) when something reminded you of a stressful experience from the past?
- Avoid thinking about or talking about a stressful experience from the past or avoid having feelings related to it?
- Avoid activities or situations because they remind you of a stressful experience from the past?
- Trouble remembering important parts of a stressful experience from the past?
- Do you have a loss of interest in things that you used to enjoy?
- Feeling distant or cut off from other people?
- Feeling emotionally numb or being unable to have loving feelings for those close to you?
- Feeling as if your future will somehow be cut short?
- Trouble falling or staying asleep?
- Feeling irritable or having angry outbursts?
- Having difficulty concentrating?
- Being "super alert" or watchful on guard?
- Feeling jumpy or easily startled?

There also were significant improvements in measures of depression, cognition, and post-concussion scores. This study and others strongly support psychostimulant use for treating PTSD with ADHD and should be considered as an effective option.

subsequently over time as his exercise had dramatically reduced, which unknowingly had been a very effective treatment for his ADHD. He developed increasing anxiety and chronic fatigue.

A psychiatrist started him on Xanax to help with anxiety but failed to see the connection between his untreated ADHD, anxiety, and chronic fatigue. His primary care doctors had referred him to specialists because the patient was worried, he had an immune problem. After all, he thought his neck lymph nodes were enlarged when he was experiencing tender points in his neck muscles, which made him feel like his nodes were swollen. He ended up getting a lymph node biopsy done, which was normal. In reality, he didn't have any problems with his lymph nodes but did have very sensitive tender points in the neck muscles that to him felt like there must be something swollen. No one told him that those tender points were part of a big picture called fibromyalgia.

While this carried on, he got increasingly frustrated. I am sure that the primary doctors he had seen were also frustrated because his tests came up normal. His fatigue had swelled to the point where he was unable to work. On the outside, he looked like a reasonably fit, healthy 27-year-old. What's a doctor to do in a situation like that? In review of his past visits with doctors, one doctor wrote in his notes that the patient was malingering, a fancy word for faking it. "There is nothing wrong; it is all in your head." I wish I could say that his story was rare, but an hour later I saw a new patient with a similar story.

Those with FM and fibromyalgia-like syndromes are metaphorically blindfolded, kidnapped, bound, and tortured with no way to protect themselves. On top of that, no one else could see what they were experiencing and thought it was all made up.

They weren't "suffering and just needed to get on with their life." I have heard the story from many patients where they did not want to disclose all the symptoms they were enduring because they previously shared them but were met with incredulous reactions.

Unfortunately, failure to connect all the dots can lead to only a partial, incomplete picture. The unfinished image tends to lead to doing more specific tests and more organ-specific treatment. Still, it fails to see all the other underlying problems with the extra-sensitive nervous system, anxiety, fibro fog, fatigue, and poor sleep.

Faces of Fibromyalgia

What are the different faces of fibromyalgia? Fibromyalgia is really on a continuum both in intensity and location of the pain. Part of the diagnosis is that it does occur in multiple regions in the body, as we discussed in previous chapters. Pain can be more intense in some areas of the body. If you have ever said, "I carry my stress in my _____," then you have, in a sense, fibromyalgia-like pain. This central pain sensitization manifests in different ways and different timelines, but there are many common themes. For many women, their first experience was severely painful periods, and as time goes on, tension headaches develop with the intensity increasing to the level of migraines. It can start to spread to other areas such as the neck, shoulders, back, and legs.

Other examples of regional fibromyalgia-like pain syndromes include irritable bowel syndrome, irritable bladder, temporomandibular disorders (TMD), chronic neck, and back pain. Multiple chemical sensitivity syndrome, female urethral syndrome, interstitial cystitis, POTS syndrome, and Gulf War syndrome all share similarities. I review these to show you how your problems are part of a bigger problem.

4. Aggravated by walking stairs or similar routine physical activity

B. During headache at least one of the two following symptoms occur:
1. Phonophobia and photophobia
2. Nausea and/or vomiting

Migraine with aura (MA) diagnostic criteria
A. At least two attacks fulfilling with at least three of the following:
1. One or more fully reversible aura symptoms indicating focal cerebral cortical and brain stem functions
2. At least one aura symptom develops gradually over more than four minutes, or two or more symptoms occur in succession
3. No aura symptom lasts more than 60 minutes; if more than one aura symptom is present, the accepted duration is proportionally increased
4. Headache follows aura with a free interval of at least 60 minutes (it may also simultaneously begin with the aura)

B. At least one of the following aura features establishes a diagnosis of migraine with typical aura:
1. Homonymous visual disturbance
2. Unilateral paresthesias and/or numbness
3. Unilateral weakness
4. Aphasia or unclassifiable speech difficulty

Notice that migraines involve amplified pain. Other people in the same room would not be feeling distressed with the volume. Also, other sensations are altered. Nausea and light sensitivity are increased. You need to be in a quiet, dark room. You will be fatigued. Relief can occur by falling asleep or taking an NSAID like ibuprofen. If taken early in the onset of symptoms, specific medications known as triptans can halt and reverse the course. Tension headaches are on a continuum and mild to moderate in nature with mild to moderate intensity. There can be light and sound sensitivity, but the levels are more tolerable.

"JT" had been doing well without any headaches. He had been very active and exercising at a very high-level during Wisconsin's warmer summers. Gradually, as it shifted into fall and winter, the weather became colder, and with other responsibilities, he wasn't able to keep up with the regular very active workouts. He started to have intermittent pressure over his face and temples. The tension spread over his sinuses. He went to the ENT doctor who treated him with steroids and antibiotics for a presumed sinus infection. He didn't improve.

Looking back at his history, he did not have sinus drainage, or congestion or cough. He also had a history of restless leg syndrome but stopped taking his gabapentin that had effectively treated his symptoms. Like many people wanting to limit medication, he had been doing better and decided to quit taking medicine. He had fared okay when he was keeping active at a very high level, but as his activity lessened, his sleep worsened, and he started developing more frequent and severe headaches. Fortunately, we were able to treat him by getting back on the gabapentin and gradually increasing his exercise. His sleep was refreshing, and his headaches improved a lot. We also needed to add duloxetine, which helped as well.

TMJ, also known as temporomandibular pain, is the pain located in the jaw and neck with a strong centralized pain component. TMJ can come on gradually or sometimes triggered by something physical such as a dental procedure or surgery or trauma. The pain is usually some achiness, throbbing type pain. A patient may have woken up from surgery with severe jaw pain that leads to heightened sensation of pain.

Intestinal Central Pain Sensitization Disorders

The most familiar is irritable bowel syndrome (IBS). There are specific criteria, but it is essential to remember that this is on a continuum. Irritable bowel involves both a heightened sensation of food traveling through the intestines and the abnormal action on the food. I like to think of IBS as a headache but located in the intestines. Both tend to have an ebb and flow with at times intense flare ups precipitated by significant stressors, poor sleep, change in exercise, or diet changes.

- **Rome criteria**. These criteria include abdominal pain and discomfort lasting on average at least one day a week in the last three months, associated with at least two of these factors: Pain and discomfort are related to defecation, and the frequency of defecation or stool consistency is altered.
- **Manning criteria**. These criteria focus on pain relief by passing stool and having incomplete bowel movements, mucus in the stool, and stool consistency changes.

The more symptoms you have, the greater the likelihood of IBS. Diagnosis is made by a careful history and sometimes tests to ensure that serious diseases are not present. In particular, inflammatory bowel diseases, celiac disease, and cancers are ruled out. Intestinal pain is caused by distention of the inside of the intestine. Think of a balloon that is inflated. As the pressure increases, alarms start to signal potential danger. After all, we don't want to have the intestines rupture as that could be deadly. People, however, with IBS, report pain at much lower levels of distention than healthy people.

Experiments using special balloons with sensors were inserted into the rectum of the study subjects. The pressure in the balloon was gradually increased until there was mild to moderate pain and then recorded. Comparisons were made between those with IBS and those without IBS. The findings showed those with IBS reported pain at about half the pressure as those without IBS.

The impact of stretching the intestines also showed different responses in the brain. Studies looking at functional MRI (fMRI) brain responses showed significant activation in the anterior insular cortex and prefrontal cortex in those with IBS vs. those without IBS. Functional magnetic resonance imaging (fMRI) is one of the imaging methods designed to assess regional changes in oxygenation and blood flow within the brain. More active areas show higher signaling.

Based on daily observation and scientific research, it is commonly known that psychological processes, both affective and cognitive, affect the functioning of the digestive system. The relation between psychological factors and visceral hypersensitivity has been implied for a long time, mainly based on studies focused on functional diseases of the digestive system.

However, until recently, the mechanism of this remained unclear, mainly due to a lack of non-invasive investigation methods. Functional brain imaging (positron emission tomography – PET, fMRI) allowed live analysis of the brain-digestive tract interaction and neurological mechanisms underlying intestinal hypersensitivity, significantly advanced research, and helped in understanding IBS. There is evidence also that increased afferent (incoming) stimulation to the brain plays a role as well.

Doctors have observed before sophisticated imaging studies were available that patients have experienced the significant effect of stress and how our thinking can affect pain and visceral response. "I am so nervous; my stomach feels so sick." There may be a reflexive response to stress with diarrhea, like dumping out something poisonous. Eating food with fiber makes a difference in the long term. Fiber is digested by good bacteria in the intestines resulting in the release of short-chain fatty acids (SCFAs). These are 2-5 carbon atoms long molecules that have many benefits. One of these, butyrate, has been shown to dampen the sensitivity of these intestinal nerves.

Functional Dyspepsia

Functional dyspepsia is a term for recurring signs and symptoms of indigestion that have no apparent cause. Signs and symptoms of functional dyspepsia may include:

- A burning sensation or discomfort in your upper abdomen or lower chest, sometimes relieved by food or antacids
- Bloating
- Belching
- An early feeling of fullness when eating
- Nausea
- "Gas pains"

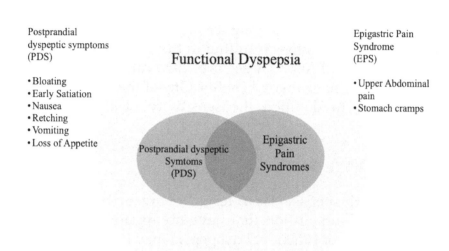

Postprandial
dyspeptic symptoms
(PDS)

Functional Dyspepsia

Epigastric Pain
Syndrome
(EPS)

• Bloating
• Early Satiation
• Nausea
• Retching
• Vomiting
• Loss of Appetite

• Upper Abdominal
pain
• Stomach cramps

Postprandial dyspeptic
Symtoms
(PDS)

Epigastric
Pain
Syndromes

Functional dyspepsia (FD) is another condition in which neuroimaging allows the analysis of dysfunctions within the brain-gut axis engaged in the processing of intestinal discomfort and pain. Patients with FD present with various abnormalities in some specific brain areas. Studies demonstrated a correlation observed between anxiety and decreased pain threshold, epigastric discomfort, burning sensation, and early satiety. Patients with functional disorders of the digestive tract are also less effective in dealing with daily-life problems. They are more inclined to be too critical of themselves, have catastrophic thoughts, or focus on their failures.

According to the recently revised Rome IV criteria, functional dyspepsia is defined by:

- Persistent or recurring dyspepsia for more than 3 months within the past 6 months
- No demonstration of a possible organic cause of the symptoms on endoscopy
- No sign that the dyspepsia is relieved only by defecation or of an association with stool irregularities.

This last criterion was introduced to rule out irritable bowel syndrome (IBS) as a possible cause of the symptoms, although around 30% of patients with functional dyspepsia also have IBS.

Comorbid psychiatric disorders, such as anxiety and depression, are prevalent in patients with gastroesophageal reflux disease (GERD) and GERD-related chest pain. Approximately 60% of GERD patients reported worsening of the symptoms during stress. Studies have used ph probes attached to the esophagus for 24 hours to measure the amount of acid present. Also, studies using manometry to assess normal pressures in the esophagus in those with GERD have been performed. Both demonstrated that the amount of acid entering the esophagus did not correlate to disease symptoms.

In other words, people with severe GERD symptoms do not necessarily have higher levels of acid in their esophagus, and those with low levels of acid do not always have fewer symptoms.

These findings suggest the influence of central pain processing on symptom perception. Stress and psychological comorbidities might predispose individuals to be more vigilant for physiological sensations, resulting in an enhanced response to a painful stimulus or a painful reaction to an innocuous stimulus may trigger or worsen chest pain of cardiac or esophageal origin.

Irritable bladder/Interstitial cystitis

Irritable bladder has been called interstitial cystitis and overactive bladder. Both involve pelvic and bladder symptoms. Typically, there is a pain in the lower pelvic region with a strong urge to urinate with at least a partial, temporary improvement in symptoms after voiding. This is felt to be a fibromyalgia-like pain disorder, but other problems can cause symptoms such as a urinary infection or cancer. A urinalysis is typically performed in addition to a careful history. Sometimes a cystoscopy looking inside the bladder or imaging studies are performed to rule out cancer.

Patients who had fibromyalgia were surveyed and filled out rating scales including Fibromyalgia Impact scores and Pelvic Floor Distress and Pelvic Urgency and Frequency. Results showed that 39% also had irritable bladder symptoms. Notice the high rates of concentration problems, which suggest a possible role of untreated ADHD.

Self-reported comorbidities

Irritable bladder or interstitial cystitis 39%,
problems with concentration 95%,
irritable bowel syndrome or GI problems 83%,
depressive symptoms 81%,
problems with balance 74%,
dry eyes/dry mouth 74%,
chronic headaches 74%,
anxiety symptoms 63%,
temporomandibular joint disorders 55%,
restless leg syndrome 55%,
chronic fatigue syndrome 56%,

Revised Fibromyalgia Impact Questionnaire
Mean FIQR= Total 57.2 (normal=<20,
Mild 20s-30s, Moderate 40-59, High>60, extreme >80)

Function score 11.2
Overall impact 15.6
Symptom score 28.2
Pain 5.5
Energy 6.7
Stiffness 6.6
Sleep 7.1
Depression 3.9
Memory problems 5.0
Anxiety 3.8
Tenderness to the touch 6.3
Balance 4.0
Sensitivity to odors and cold bright, light, loudness noise 6.5

The majority (93%) of women indicated that they experience bladder or pelvic pain occasionally, with more than half reporting that they experience discomfort regularly. Higher FIQR scores positively correlated with higher pelvic floor distress and urinary urgency scores (PUF), indicating that there is an increased presence and severity of urinary and pelvic floor distress symptoms among those with a more severe FM. This is interesting because only 39% self-report a diagnosis of irritable/pain bladder or interstitial cystitis. Perhaps non-urogynecologic providers are less confident in diagnosing specific bladder disorders.

Often the chief complaint someone has directs which doctor you go to first. If you have neck and back pain, you may end up in an orthopedic surgeon's office compared to someone whose primary symptoms are pelvic pain and urinary symptoms. The orthopedic surgeon is unlikely to ask, let alone diagnose other pain disorders. A patient likely has had these symptoms for years and has normalized the symptoms and may be less likely to bring up the signs to their internist or family practice doctor.

Vulvodynia

Vulvodynia, pain with normal pressure on the vulva, also is related to fibromyalgia. The vulvodynia's criteria included having had more than three months of vulvar discomfort, located at the opening of the vagina, that has not resolved. Symptoms can range from mild discomfort to severe and debilitating pain. It may be only in one area, or it may move around. It may be sharp or diffuse, and it may come and go. Symptoms include burning, stinging, rawness, itching, throbbing, and overall soreness.

Vulvodynia can cause pain during sexual intercourse, exercise, sitting, and other aspects of daily function. Vulvodynia is associated with other chronic comorbid pain conditions such as fibromyalgia, interstitial cystitis, and irritable bowel syndrome. The presence of vulvodynia or any of the other comorbid pain conditions increases the likelihood that a woman will have one or more of the other chronic pain conditions.

Dysmenorrhea and endometriosis also appear to have central pain sensitization problems. Similar research has demonstrated that those with endometriosis have altered responses to pain seen on functional MRIs. There are different levels of excitatory chemicals in areas of the brain that are involved in managing pain.

Take-home points:
- **Central sensitization and pain amplification are common threads with multiple chronic pain disorders.**

- **These disorders commonly occur together.**
- **Fibromyalgia-like pain disorders are real and prevalent.**

Chronic Back Pain/Failed Back Surgery Syndrome

Failed back surgery syndrome (FBSS) is a term used to describe a clinical entity that has been acknowledged since the advent of spinal surgery. A more functional definition is "when the outcome of lumbar spinal surgery does not meet the pre-surgical expectations of the patient and surgeon." In other words, you don't have significant improvement in back pain after surgery. Failure rates of spinal surgery in the literature range between 10% and 40%. Conservatively, we might assume a failure rate of 20%. This is similar to the outcomes in knee replacement and hip replacement surgeries.

Could the failed back surgery syndrome be part of the fibromyalgia continuum?

This hypothesis was put to the test in a study comparing fibromyalgia and failed back surgery syndrome patients (FBSS) to see if there is a common central pain sensitivity syndrome pathology. They demonstrated that the variables of familial, symptomatological, and psychological makeup of people were very similar. FM and FBSS can be looked at as the same problem. Surgery might be avoided in those with FM and focus on treatment with a more comprehensive approach, as will be discussed later.

Gulf War Illness

A prominent condition affecting Gulf War veterans is a cluster of medically unexplained chronic symptoms that can include fatigue, headaches, joint pain, indigestion, insomnia, dizziness, respiratory disorders, and memory problems.

Gulf War Illness (GWI) has developed in 25% to 32% of the 697,000 US military personnel deployed to the Persian Gulf in 1990 to 1991. The rate in non-deployed forces may have been 15%. Two sets of criteria have been used to define symptoms. In 1998, the CDC proposed the Chronic Multi-symptom Illness (CMI) criteria that defined cases by having ≥1 chronic symptom from at least 2 of 3 categories (musculoskeletal pain, fatigue, mood-cognition).

The 2000 Kansas criteria were based on symptoms that were significantly more prevalent in deployed than non-deployed personnel.

Cases were defined by having symptoms in at least 3 of 6 categories:
- musculoskeletal pain,
- neurological/cognitive/mood,
- fatigue/sleep,
- respiratory,
- gastrointestinal, and
- skin problems.

A study looked to see if Gulf war illness shared many of fibromyalgia and chronic fatigue characteristics. Were these the same problems with different names? GWI, Chronic fatigue syndrome (CFS), and CFS/FM had equivalent scores for the nine Chronic Fatigue Syndrome Symptom Severity questionnaire items. These included equal scores in the level of fatigue, cognition, muscle pain, headache, sleep, and exertional exhaustion.

Measurements of pain on trigger points known as dolorimetry were analyzed among the CFS, FM, and GWI and compared to healthy sedentary controls. They wanted to see if they shared hyperalgesia, the increased level of pain at lower pressure thresholds. They found a shared overlapping shift of pain reported at low levels among those with CFS, FM, and GWI.

Evaluation of fatigue was used with the multidimensional fatigue inventory domain, a comprehensive assessment of fatigue and related issues. General tiredness, physical fatigue, reduced activity, and reduced motivation were similarly higher in those with GWI, CFS, and FM. Gulf War Syndrome which had been a mystery but is probably under the umbrella of fibromyalgia. It is likely that "COVID long-haul syndrome" will also be linked to fibromyalgia, but time and more research will tell.

GWI, CFS, and FM appear to be similar faces of the same underlying problem.

Chapter 6
"Fibro Fog"

Fibro fog refers to general cognitive difficulties, which include fatigue, decreased motivation, low energy, poor concentration, reduced alertness, and forgetfulness. Mental symptoms can be more disturbing than widespread pain. They can change the lives of people suffering, sometimes dramatically so. Whereas widespread musculoskeletal pain, tenderness, and fatigue may be the hallmark symptoms of fibromyalgia, patients rank "fibro fog" as highly distressing.

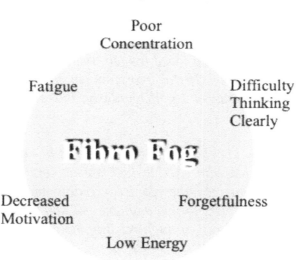

The cause of "fibro fog" has been studied and has shown interesting findings. There is a connection between ADHD, chronic fatigue syndrome, and fibromyalgia. A study published in 2018 in the journal <u>Pain Medicine</u> looked at the frequency of ADHD in those who had fibromyalgia. They discovered that nearly half of patients with fibromyalgia also had ADHD. Those who had ADHD and fibromyalgia were

10.6 times more likely to report cognitive impairment in their thinking and remembering. In the combined group, 91% reported anxiety, markedly more than the FM alone group.

The take-home points of the study are that ADHD should be considered for those with FM because it is often unrecognized and can have a significant impact on functioning in those with fibromyalgia.

"Hal" came to see me because of fatigue and was wondering if he should get his testosterone checked and if he had any vitamin deficiencies. He reported very nonspecific fatigue. Hal didn't have any shortness of breath with exercise. However, he didn't always feel the motivation or enthusiasm to do things. He was in his 50s and was currently working in sales, which he changed to more because of the significant increase in pay he was offered. Previously he had worked in tool and die and loved his job. It was very hands-on, and he was always moving. In his free time in his 20s and 30s, he enjoyed playing softball and golf regularly, but as he got older, he became less active.

In high school, he did "okay" and was told that he could have better grades if he applied himself. He had always preferred hands-on learning and seldom read the required reading but instead would read summary notes. He, to this day, has not done much reading. If he has to learn something through reading, he will have to reread it multiple times to retain it.

Fast forward to his current job, where he is much less active. It is more stressful because he has to sit and go through emails and reports that he doesn't enjoy. He has had to learn new technology and often experiences a sense of feeling overwhelmed with those aspects of his job. He does enjoy talking with clients and would go back to working tool and die if it were not for the significant reduction in income.

I took a careful history and physical exam and did blood work. He had a normal blood chemistry panel, testosterone level, thyroid panel, and complete blood count. He also had a normal sleep study done. He had mildly elevated blood pressure and moderately high cholesterol. He was about 50 lbs. above where he weighed many years ago when he was working as a tool and die worker and exercising regularly. He also reported having chronic neck and back pain, intermittent headaches, abdominal bloating, and leg pain.

I performed the WHO adult ADHD screening questionnaire, which showed his levels to be in the range highly probable for ADHD. This revelation started the conversation about the connection between untreated ADHD and fatigue. Let's learn more about chronic fatigue, fibromyalgia-like pain, and ADHD.

Chronic Fatigue Syndrome (CFS)

Chronic Fatigue Syndrome (CFS) affects millions of people each year. Although it is often perceived to be a disorder characterized by only long-term, persistent fatigue that cannot be explained by another medical condition or by ongoing exertion. A variety of other symptoms are typically present for at least six months. These additional symptoms include post-exertion malaise, muscle, and joint pain, headaches, unrefreshing sleep, tender areas, and pain in the neck. For some patients, the most distressing symptoms of CFS are executive functioning deficits that include impaired short-term memory, delayed reaction time, and a subjective sensation of "mental fogginess." Combined with fatigue and pain, these executive function deficits can be debilitating. It is estimated that they affect as many as 80% of all individuals who suffer from CFS.

A variety of treatment options are available to patients with CFS, but none have proven to be universally useful. Among these options are cognitive-behavioral therapy, exercise therapy, dietary interventions, homeopathic treatments, and pharmacological interventions. The symptoms resonate with the mental struggles of fibromyalgia. That begs the question.

Is ADHD a big part of CFS?

Many feel that Chronic Fatigue Syndrome (CFS) is on the spectrum of fibromyalgia. However, CFS has more emphasis on fatigue and cognitive symptoms. Research has shown ADHD and ADHD symptoms are common in both.

What if patients with CFS were treated with a stimulant?

That hypothesis was put to the test in a study that was designed primarily to determine whether a common psychostimulant medication lisamphetamine (LDX) known also by the brand name Vyvanse could be used to reduce executive functioning deficits in CFS patients who also present with clinically significant executive functioning deficits. It also measured reductions in fatigue and pain with treatment vs. placebo.

Relative to participants in the placebo group, those in the LDX group had less fatigue, less pain, higher overall functioning, and fewer ADHD symptoms at the end of the trial compared to baseline. There were improvements measured globally, but there were specific measures I wanted to highlight.

Higher scores mean increased functioning. Compared to the placebo score of 1, the LDX score went to 21 for working memory. It was 3 in the placebo group compared to 14 for the organization of material, and very interestingly, it was 3.8 compared to 23 for initiation. The difficulties with self-initiation are something I have observed clinically. This is a common frustration for those with untreated ADHD and shows up in many ways.

A student delays getting started on researching and writing a paper. An adult wants to lose weight and eat healthier but gets caught in unfulfilled intentions and goals. "I know I should make a meal plan before I go shopping. I should go to the store and only get what is on the list. When I get home, I should take the time to cook and clean up after the meal."

A recent patient achieved the first step purchasing the ingredients for a healthy meal, but when she got home, she felt overwhelmed and wanted to just order out pickup from a restaurant rather than take the time to prepare the food. It is like the student who remembers to take their assignment sheet and homework home but then decides to play video games or watch TV instead. Treatment of ADHD allows for the follow through on the good intentions by removing the distracting barriers that would hijack his or her well laid plans.

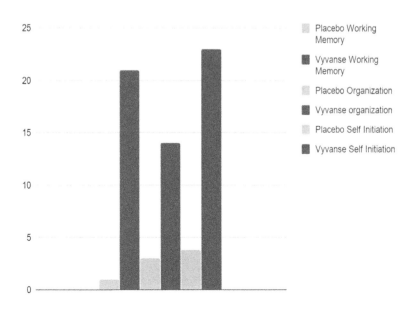

A recent patient had boxes in his garage containing papers that were left over from a previous job that were sitting in his garage for many years. He had always had intentions to get through it and knew most of it was meaningless and he could throw it away, but he had a hard time getting started. With treatment for ADHD, he was able to filter through the boxes and keep the few papers he treasured and throw the rest away. For others, it could simply be getting projects started at home without having to be prodded to get them done. Many with chronic fatigue syndrome have difficulty with these tasks and likely are from untreated and diagnosed ADHD.

ADHD and Chronic Fatigue Syndrome

Is ADHD the linchpin of the cognitive component of fibromyalgia?

Is Chronic Fatigue Syndrome part of the continuum of fibromyalgia with these patients having ADHD predominantly inattentive type?

The research points in that direction.

Chapter 7
ADHD

My first exposure to ADHD was in a talk on it during my first year in medical school in 1992. I held skepticism of the disorder and thought it was just an excuse for kids who couldn't behave. Was it just a rationalization for children's underperformance? My view changed over time starting with my combined residency in pediatrics and internal medicine from 1996-2000. All my experience and training on ADHD was in the pediatric clinic. None of the physicians ever brought it up during the care and management of my adult patients. I saw the improvement in the function of the children I treated.

Combining the learning of 2 residencies that would separately take 3 years each to complete into 6 years is a lot to cover. The combined program accomplished it in 4 years and allowed great training. Management of asthma, for example, in children and adults was very similar with dosing differences for medications. Similarly, the understanding of ADHD and FM would turn out to have common underlying issues that applied to children and adults. However, ADHD has been commonly thought of as a pediatric problem and FM has been more recognized in adults.

The reasons I decided to do a combined residency is because I liked using medical science and wanted to have an in-depth understanding of the nonsurgical care of children and adults. Some residents will decide to go on to a fellowship in specialized health problems such as cardiology and gastroenterology. I, however, didn't want to limit my care to specific symptoms and organs and relatively ignore the rest of the body. I wanted to take a holistic, whole body, approach to caring for my patients.

After residency I started my practice in pediatrics and internal medicine (non-operative care of adults). I continued to want to learn and grow in my understanding of health problems. I was told by a physician mentor during my premedical college program called Target MD that every 7 years half of what you learn in medicine changes. That surprised me, but since then, this revelation has repeated itself in many areas over and over.

Until the late 1990s we didn't realize that H. Pylori bacteria was the cause of most stomach ulcers. I remember learning this and sharing it with my senior resident during my surgery rotation. He was initially incredulous as he never heard of that before. Another example of how management changes is the use of a medication called carvedilol, a type of beta blocker, for the treatment of heart failure. It had previously thought that you should never use a beta blocker to treat heart failure, but studies had shown clear benefits and changed the management of heart failure.

I had always been interested in helping the most people possible. The biggest killer of men and women is heart disease. I had observed that a lot of people were dying with heart disease who, according to guidelines, would have been told that they were "ok." It didn't really hit me until around 2004, at the age of 33, that I started to understand the heart disease mystery more in-depth. I had up to that point had a cholesterol of 167, and LDL of 113 and an HDL of 30. All of these are in the low-risk range. I had been exercising regularly and eating a pretty good diet. I didn't smoke and had a normal blood pressure. There was a clinical lipidologist who had started practicing in the area and was doing more advanced lipid testing. I was previously very skeptical of the advanced testing and thought it was unnecessary. I thought I had all the understanding of the tests needed to properly assess for the risk of developing a heart attack or stroke.

A representative of the NMR lipoprofile company had offered to do a free profile. He shared my results which showed my LDL particles to be at 2100, in the very high range. He said he can't give me medical advice but told me I should see the same lipidologist who I previously had been skeptical of. I got a heart scan showing a small amount of plaque in my heart arteries. Two additional blood tests, an hsCRP (*a measure of inflammation and heart risk*) and lipoprotein a (*a protein that attaches to bad cholesterol and increases heart risk*) were elevated. My skepticism changed to gratitude. I was humbled and thankful. My interest in lipidology was piqued, so I pursued advanced training and certification by becoming a diplomat of the Board of Clinical Lipidology.

My progression in cholesterol and heart disease management is similar to the growth in my understanding of ADHD, especially ADHD in adults. Many with the condition are skeptical of the very problem they have, mainly due to a misunderstanding. I have found how the treatment of adults and children with ADHD could have very positive impacts and change the course of one's life.

In the early 2000s, I started to read more about ADHD and how what was previously thought of as a mainly pediatric problem that usually never went away and continued into adulthood. I had a rare recent patient who was prompted to see me as a friend of his because of my expertise in cholesterol management and interest in healthy eating. He was rare because he was diagnosed in the 1960s with "ADHD" due to his extreme hyperactivity.

He was treated with methylphenidate and did well but then at age 17 the pediatrician stopped it. He was told he didn't need it anymore as he was an adult. On further history taking, like most adults, it didn't magically go away, and he continued to have ADHD into adulthood that was unrecognized and unmanaged leading to impairment. His adult daughter also had symptoms but had never been identified.

My first adult patient I treated had started with the care of his son who was struggling with what turned out to be ADHD. The father reported having ADHD symptoms just like his son's while he was in elementary school and now continued to struggle in adult life. I treated him, somewhat nervously, as I had never treated an adult with ADHD. He responded well, just like his son. I started to become more aware of my own blind spot of adult ADHD. I started using the World Health Organization ADHD screening along with a history to diagnose and then treat more and more adults. I also continued to treat my pediatric patients as they reached adulthood. I started seeing family members of those with ADHD. Why wait until adulthood before treating the problem?

The following image illustrates the Adult Self-Report Scale-V1.1 (ASRS-V1.1). The questionnaire is used as a starting point to evaluate a patient's signs and symptoms that can be indicative of Adult ADHD. The screening questions are intended for people aged 18 years or older. See the Appendix on page 251 for a chart that you, or your patient, can complete.

Adult Self-Report Scale-V1.1 (ASRS-V1.1)

Adult Self-Report Scale-V1.1 (ASRS-V1.1) Screener
from WHO Composite International Diagnostic Interview

	Date					
		Never	Rarely	Sometimes	Often	Very Often

Check the box that best describes how you have felt and conducted yourself over the past 6 months. Please give the completed questionnaire to your healthcare professional during your next appointment to discuss the results.

1. How often do you have trouble wrapping up the final details of a project, once the challenging parts have been done?

2. How often do you have difficulty getting things in order when you have to do a task that requires organization?

3. How often do you have problems remembering appointments or obligations?

4. When you have a task that requires a lot of thought, how often do you avoid or delay getting started?

5. How often do you fidget or squirm with your hands or feet when you have to sit down for a long time?

6. How often do you feel overly active and compelled to do things, like you were driven by a motor?

Add the number of checkmarks that appear in the darkly shaded area. Four (4) or more checkmarks indicate that your symptoms may be consistent with Adult ADHD. It may be beneficial for you to talk with your healthcare provider about an evaluation.

The 6-question Adult Self-Report Scale Version 1.1 (ASRS-V1.1) Screener is a subset of the WHO's 18-question Adult ADHD Self-Report Scale Version 1.1 (Adult ASRS v1.1) Symptom Checklist.

ATZ9241 PRINTED IN USA. J6R0434361MC600 ASRS v1.1 Screener COPYRIGHT © 2003 World Health Organization (WHO). Reprinted with permission of WHO. All rights reserved.

In similar ways, doctors regularly screen for depression, high cholesterol, alcoholism, smoking, and diabetes among other diseases. These issues can have profound impacts on overall health. Typically, someone struggling with these doesn't come in and directly say I have diabetes or have lots of plaque in my arteries. They also don't say "I have alcohol problems and am severely depressed." Neither will they usually say I have FM or ADHD. These problems become normalized into the fabric of their life. All of these issues are profoundly impactful on one's health. All of these can be effectively managed and treated.

Because these problems may be less apparent, we screen for them. Heart disease is silent, so we screen for it by looking for high blood pressure, diabetes, and high cholesterol. I perform advanced lipid testing because awareness can lead to early treatment and can prevent and even reverse heart disease. A very powerful and effective group of medicines called statins greatly reduce risk of a heart attack or stroke. However, research showed the limits of the very effective statins, as it didn't prevent all heart attacks. Many taking them still were having heart attacks. What other effective options were available as other medicines such as niacin, which had shown some preliminary benefits, but when added to a statin didn't reduce the risk of a heart attack?

I learned the powerful effect of a whole-foods plant-based diet from my wife who was doing continuing education and had recommended I read the book, *The China Study*, by T. Colin Campbell. I did further in-depth research and was convinced of the benefits of a whole-foods plant-based diet. I started implementing it for myself and then for my patients. If I couldn't eat that way, it would be hypocritical for me to seriously recommend it and be able to effectively guide people as they embark on what many might consider a radical diet change. You will learn more about the role of diet in the chapters on treatment.

Similarly, I learned the significant struggles adults with untreated ADHD very often endured. Comorbidities will occur in most adults with ADHD at some point in their lives. Comorbidities are health problems that commonly occur with another problem. Treatment alone with medications can have great benefits, but many also need lifestyle coaching to help get through their problems. The medication moors patients so they can benefit from the coaching and implementation of lifestyle changes.

There are many of the struggles we have talked about in fibromyalgia and related pain disorders that also have ADHD. Treatment of ADHD plays an important role. However, adult ADHD awareness in physicians and therapists is often underappreciated. It is often overlooked and diagnosed as anxiety, depression, or personality disorders.

ADHD, especially in adults, is a lot like fibromyalgia; it is often overlooked and misunderstood. There also is a big stigma attached to it for many, including physicians. Most people, including physicians, recognize depression as a valid mental health issue. Still, acceptance of ADHD is not as common in adults. This is not surprising because it takes about 17 years for medical advances to become routinely implemented in practice. Advanced lipid testing for heart disease is being used by more physicians as awareness has increased.

Still, routine screening of children for the development of heart disease with a simple cholesterol panel is not routinely implemented despite multiple studies demonstrating the effectiveness and preventing the development of heart disease in adulthood. Heart disease has far less of a stigma than ADHD and fibromyalgia. This stigma is an important reason diagnosis and management have been delayed.

The consequences of the factors that lead to heart disease can be very deadly and disabling. ADHD also occurs commonly in fibromyalgia and chronic pain disorders. Similar to how treating depression leads to healthier outcomes, so too does treatment of ADHD. My hope is that this chapter will give greater perspective into a condition that affects so many and quietly causes so much suffering. This condition also occurs at much higher rates in those with fibromyalgia, chronic fatigue syndrome among other fibromyalgia-like pain syndromes. Treatment for ADHD has reduced symptoms in these syndromes and has improved overall functioning in multiple areas.

What are the consequences of untreated ADHD?

ADHD affects nearly 8 million American adults and can lead to increased healthcare costs, higher divorce rates, unemployment and motor vehicle accidents. Mortality rates are 4 times greater in adults with untreated ADHD. "For too long, the validity of ADHD as a medical disorder has been challenged," the investigators write. "Policy makers should take heed of these data and allocate a fair share of healthcare and research resources to people with ADHD."

"For clinicians, early identification and treatment should become the rule rather than the exception."

Yet, the vast majority of these patients remain undiagnosed, with only one quarter seeking medical help for impairment associated with ADHD. Even those patients who seek help often aren't identified as having ADHD. Women with ADHD have lifelong struggles, and their symptoms affect every aspect of their lives. Women with ADHD often have children with ADHD, a difficult undertaking in the best of circumstances. There are special challenges balancing home, work, and intimacy. Untreated ADHD has higher rates of addictions which can have major health consequences. The most common and socially acceptable is food addictions and unhealthy eating, along with tobacco use, and alcohol in addition to cocaine and marijuana use at higher levels.

Treatment of ADHD can help battle these issues much more effectively. Is treating children with ADHD with stimulants helpful, harmful, or neutral? A study followed boys into adulthood to look at the difference in development of subsequent psychiatric diagnosis including depression and anxiety. They discovered that treatment had a profound effect of protecting from depression. Put another way, not treating ADHD puts someone a much greater risk of anxiety, depression, oppositional defiant disorder, bipolar disorder, and repeating a grade in school, among others.

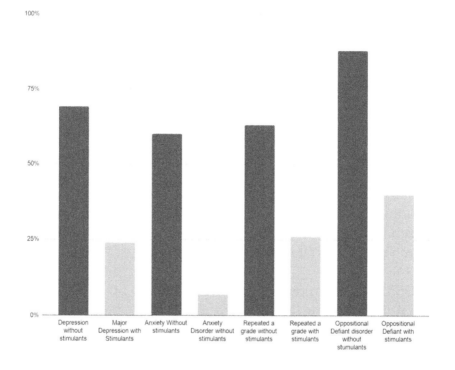

For all the concern about side effects of treating ADHD, more emphasis should be placed on the consequences of not treating and the benefits of treating. This applies to multiple areas in addition to fibromyalgia and fibromyalgia related disorders.

What is ADHD?

ADHD is a neurobiological condition that often starts in childhood and involves impairing symptoms of inattention, hyperactivity, and impulsivity. People with the disorder characteristically have difficulty in persistence towards goals, tasks, and the future in general. They are distracted from achieving their goal by irrelevant distractions. Like fibromyalgia and depression, ADHD diagnosis is made through a careful history of listening to past and current difficulties.

There are no specific tests such as blood work or imaging studies to make the diagnosis, but psychometric tools like the World Health Organization ADHD adult assessment and other rating scales are typically used. Functional MRIs have shown differences in brain processes in those with ADHD, especially involving the part of the brain known as the prefrontal cortex. At this point, fMRIs are only used in research and are unlikely to be used diagnostically. The research reinforces the neurobiological cause of ADHD.

The DSM V (Diagnostic Statistical Manual 5th edition), the manual for making psychiatric diagnoses, has criteria for ADHD in children and adults.

Core Symptoms of ADHD

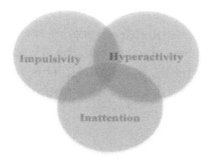

How Is It Diagnosed?
DSM-5 Criteria

A valid neuro-developmental disorder involving:
Inattention Symptoms (5 of 9)

Often:

- fails to give close attention to details
- difficulty sustaining attention
- does not seem to listen
- does not follow through on instructions
- difficulty organizing tasks or activities
- avoids tasks requiring sustained mental effort
- loses things necessary for tasks
- easily distracted
- forgetful in daily activities

DSM-5 Criteria for ADHD

People with ADHD show a persistent pattern of inattention and/or hyperactivity-impulsivity that interferes with functioning or development:

Inattention: Six or more symptoms of inattention for children up to age 16 years, or five or more for adolescents age 17 years and older and adults; symptoms of inattention have been present for at least 6 months, and they are inappropriate for developmental level:

- *Often fails to give close attention to details or makes careless mistakes in schoolwork, at work, or with other activities.*
- *Often has trouble holding attention on tasks or play activities.*
- *Often does not seem to listen when spoken to directly.*

- *Often does not follow through on instructions and fails to finish schoolwork, chores, or duties in the workplace (e.g., loses focus, side-tracked).*
- *Often has trouble organizing tasks and activities.*
- *Often avoids, dislikes, or is reluctant to do tasks that require mental effort over a long period of time (such as schoolwork or homework).*
- *Often loses things necessary for tasks and activities (e.g., school materials, pencils, books, tools, wallets, keys, paperwork, eyeglasses, mobile telephones).*
- *Is often easily distracted*
- *Is often forgetful in daily activities.*

Hyperactivity and Impulsivity: Six or more symptoms of hyperactivity-impulsivity for children up to age 16 years, or five or more for adolescents age 17 years and older and adults; symptoms of hyperactivity-impulsivity have been present for at least six months to an extent that is disruptive and inappropriate for the person's developmental level:

- *Often fidgets with or taps hands or feet or squirms in the seat.*
- *Often leaves a seat in situations when remaining seated is expected.*
- *Often runs about or climbs in situations where it is not appropriate (adolescents or adults may be limited to feeling restless).*
- *Often unable to play or take part in leisure activities quietly.*
- *Is often "on the go" acting as if "driven by a motor."*
- *Often talks excessively.*
- *Often blurts out an answer before a question has been completed.*
- *Often has trouble waiting for their turn.*
- *Often interrupts or intrudes on others (e.g., butts into conversations or games)*

for your intelligence. ADHD typically occurs in families similar to other medical problems like diabetes and high cholesterol. If a parent has it, there is about a 50% chance their child has it.

Most parents and grandparents have never been diagnosed, but this can be an epiphany for many as they look back at their life. With the insight, there is a bittersweet satisfaction for finally having a diagnosis that connects these before unconnected dots. There also can be one of sadness and frustration for never being diagnosed and treated earlier in their life.

"Earl" was diagnosed with ADHD by me in his late 60s after being his doctor for many years. He had intermittent brief success with dietary adherence and diabetic control following a whole-food plant-based diet. Earl knew what to do but continually made impulsive food decisions and snacked throughout the day even though he wasn't really hungry and had a relatively sedentary lifestyle. The food choices also were the calorie dense, nutritionally depleted foods of the standard American diet. He was poor at planning and initiating healthy food choices, leaving him even more vulnerable to fast food options and stress eating.

This sparked the possibility that maybe he had ADHD that I had previously overlooked. I asked him about his academic history. He told me that his high school guidance counselor said he would be lucky to graduate high school, let alone college due to academic difficulties. He pushed hard through college and found a career as a social worker, which he enjoyed working with disadvantaged boys. He enjoyed talking and social interaction with them. He, however, struggled in other ways and was now having an impact on his ability to control his diabetes.

Further testing with WHO adult ADHD questionnaire showed his scores to be in the ADHD range. He was treated with methylphenidate and came back at his next visits with tears. "I know I wasn't stupid, but I always felt I was because I would struggle with retaining what I read and focusing on tasks. Now, I can perform my job so much better and am able to adhere much more effectively to eating a plant-based diet and haven't been stress eating." Treatment allowed him to adhere to a whole-food plant-based diet with seemingly less effort, similar to a student who now goes from getting Cs to As when their ADHD is treated. His diabetes control responded, as well. His weight came down, and he felt better.

I also see this in those with ADHD who smoke. Smokers, like other addictions, occur much more commonly in those with untreated ADHD. They want to quit smoking for good reasons, but they struggle with life and the effects of untreated ADHD. They know they would be much healthier if they stop but struggle to do so. Treatment of the ADHD levels the playing field. It takes a barrier away similar to how glasses allow someone to see the baseball better and be able to hone his skills to hit the baseball more effectively.

ADHD usually is present in many other psychiatric disorders, in addition to other medical problems. About 50% of adults with anxiety disorders and 33% with depression have ADHD. About 1/3 of men with alcohol dependence and 28% with drug dependence have ADHD.

There are differences between those with ADHD alone and those with coexisting conditions. Those with ADHD and depression are more frequently depressed and moody. With anxiety, they are more likely to panic over not performing well in school or work or with losing items. They are more likely to self-describe themselves in self-deprecating ways. Those with ADHD and learning disorders are more likely, but not always, to have particular trouble with math or reading skills along with inattention. Those with ADHD alone are more likely to substitute calorie dense nutritionally deficient food, caffeine, and nicotine for healthy ways of coping with stress. Many struggle with binge eating disorder.

In contrast, those with a substance use disorder actively seek out illicit substances to the point of interfering with daily functioning. The use of food to cope with anxiety is most common and can impair functioning as well. Nearly half of severely obese people have ADHD. Treatment of binge eating disorder has been shown to help reduce impulsive eating and help organize their meal planning better with better adherence.

Contrary to some people's concerns that treatment with psychostimulants increases the risk of substance use through treatment with ADHD with stimulants, ADHD does not increase the risk of developing substance use disorders but is protective against it. Stimulant treatment of ADHD appears to reduce the risk of substance use disorders by 50%. Those with untreated ADHD are 3-4 times more likely to develop some kind of addiction in an attempt to self-regulate.

Chronic fatigue syndrome has many of the same clinical symptoms as fibromyalgia. Many feel it falls on the fibromyalgia spectrum. Studies have shown that those who had chronic fatigue syndrome and ADHD had more severe anxiety and depression symptoms. It was found that depressive symptoms and ADHD severity were significant predictors of fatigue intensity. The group with ADHD had a 62% rate of fatigue, much more than the frequency in healthy adults. The relationship between depression and fibromyalgia is highly complex. Are you depressed because you are in pain? It is sometimes unclear which came first, but they are related and self-perpetuating.

Most adults, 90-95%, with ADHD have never been diagnosed or had been in childhood and are not being treated. Many adults may have camouflaged their primarily inattentive symptoms. Many cases in adults go unrecognized or are seen by physicians that are not familiar with the subtleties of adult ADHD. This missed diagnosis applies to fibromyalgia as well.

The case of Marilyn, taken from a case report by Dr. Joel Young, a psychiatrist in Michigan who has done extensive research and writing on adolescents and adults with ADHD, is enlightening. Her story demonstrates some of these essential features and may resonate with you or someone you know.

She had been diagnosed with fibromyalgia for four years and had a history of carpal tunnel and irritable bowel syndrome (IBS). Despite being treated with pain medicines, she continued to have generalized pain. She also had been very frustrated with difficulty reading, forgetting to return phone calls, and missing appointments. She frequently missed portions of conversations and had a hard time following plot lines during movies.

Her primary care doctor also was frustrated because, despite numerous referrals to specialists to help her, she still struggled. Her workup was negative, except for having multiple trigger points on the exam. She had been to counseling and tried various antidepressants with mild stabilization of depression symptoms, but no meaningful improvement to fatigue and pain.

Her family history included a brother who had a high aptitude but never graduated high school and two children treated for ADHD since grade school. Her mother had chronic depression and had received electroconvulsive therapy 30 years earlier. Through history and standardized checklists, she was diagnosed with ADHD and started on long-acting Adderall 10mg. The dose was adjusted up to 20 mg XR every AM.

A month later, at her next visit, she had increased wakefulness, and ability to focus on reading and details of daily living. She subsequently reported more energy, less depression, and functional and social improvement. Her pain symptoms remitted. She stated, "without Adderall XR, I feel overwhelmed and tense. My muscles seem so tight. On the medication, I function so much better." Her need for pain medicine diminished, as did her reliance on physical therapy. Three years later, she had sustained her improvements.

This story reflects everyday experiences he and his colleagues have had at their clinic managing patients with fibromyalgia and ADHD. In their study on the effect of treating ADHD in those with fibromyalgia they found that seventy percent of the patients with fibromyalgia had ADHD.

At a basic level, ADHD interrupts the brain's ability to filter out extraneous stimuli. Physical and psychological sensations can overwhelm and can create intolerance to what non-ADHD brains can comfortably handle. ADHD medications work by enhancing filtering ability so that pain is noticed less and increasing attention to other behaviors that can "distract" from underlying pain. This process is similar to how physical activity tends to "distract" from the underlying pain by requiring careful focus to the task at hand. It is common in patients with fibromyalgia-like pain to report they don't notice the pain when they are physically busy.

The most effective medications are psychostimulants. They work by increasing the levels of dopamine and to an extent norepinephrine. Less effective medications include amotaxafine and bupropion.

Take-home Points:
- Attention-deficit/hyperactivity disorder (ADHD) is an underdiagnosed, undertreated, and often comorbid and debilitating condition in adults.
- Effective treatment of adult ADHD improves symptoms, emotional lability, and patient functioning, often leading to favorable outcomes, such as safer driving and reduced criminality.
- Physicians should familiarize themselves with ADHD symptoms in adults to diagnose and manage ADHD and comorbidities appropriately in these patients.
- A complicating, predisposing factor that may contribute to the onset, persistence, and exacerbation of FM symptoms, implicates enhanced attention (hypervigilance) to pain-related information.
- ADHD is considered the Diabetes of psychiatry because it is connected to so many other psychiatric conditions. It is also the most easily treatable psychiatric condition.

Studies in chronic pain patients suggest that greater attention to pain signals in combination with the preoccupation with pain at the expense of other environmental information correlates with higher pain intensity and pain amplification, experienced in more body areas of pain. These results correspond with data of examinations in FM patients investigating the role of attention. The FM patients displayed an exaggerated focus on painful body signals but not on non-noxious somatosensory signals than rheumatoid patients and healthy controls. These findings indicate that hypervigilance was related to pain-related fear and catastrophizing, suggesting that they are intrinsically linked. Both are associated with heightened attentional vigilance to pain.

Unfortunately, just as with fibromyalgia, doctors don't often consider ADHD in their list of possible causes, also known as differential diagnoses. Differential diagnoses are the list of all medical diseases and disorders that could explain a patient's symptoms. We generally group them by organ system. Unfortunately, ADHD and fibromyalgia-like disorders have symptoms that cover every organ system. The more organ systems, the greater the list of potential sub-specialists a patient may see.

Someone may enter the system with severe sinus pain thinking they have another sinus infection but are having a sinus migraine without an infection. The physician might not cast a broader net to elicit the chronic diffuse pain that he also has been struggling with. We will talk more about that in the chapters on manifestations of fibromyalgia-like disorders. Still, it is vital to recognize the difficulties physicians have to make a careful diagnosis for now.

Sometimes physicians may feel pressured for time. It may seem unrelated to the immediate concern, and it is much easier just to prescribe antibiotics that worked in the past. The antibiotic likely didn't have much of a role as the sinus migraine is self-limited to a few hours to a couple of days and would have improved on its own.

With those suffering from unknown and untreated ADHD and pain, especially in adults, they usually do not come in thinking they have ADHD. They more often present with other symptoms such as anxiety, palpitations, and panic attacks. They may feel general fatigue. They may have diffuse body pain or pain in regional locations of the body, such as lower back pain or irritable bowel syndrome. They may have migraine headaches or abdominal pain. Like other disorders, ADHD can be viewed on a continuum from mild to severe, similar to diabetes or high blood pressure.

Spectrum of Fibromyalgia Symptoms

Mild   Moderate   Severe

The following are reasons for adult ADHD misdiagnosis and missed diagnosis.

- "It is just a pediatric problem, and they will likely outgrow it." Studies show ADHD is present in about 5% of adults. I recently had a 19-year-old patient who came in during the COVID epidemic with chest pain. On further evaluation, he had a history of mild autism, ADHD, and mood disorder. The psychiatrist who was managing his meds decided he no longer needed the Vyvanse to treat the ADHD and stopped it. He didn't place him on an alternative stimulant. The thought was he didn't need it anymore because he was not in school. Within a week of stopping it, he developed progressive pain in his neck, shoulders, jaw, and chest.

  On exam, he was exquisitely tender in the classic fibromyalgia tender points, with the remainder of his exam being normal. Before coming in, he had asked the psychiatrist if any of his new meds for his mood disorder could be causing pain and was told that none of them did. A review of his meds showed that they were unlikely to provoke chest pain. However, the removal of his Vyvanse and his new, more restricted exercise due to COVID, likely were the causes of the new pain.

- Some physicians are still skeptical of the diagnoses and think it could be a conspiracy that pharmaceutical companies schemed to create a disorder to sell medications.
- Physicians that care for adults are unlikely to have had much training, if any, at all in diagnosing and treating ADHD.

In a survey of primary care physicians who had reported having at least 30 patients a week with ADHD, anxiety, depression, generalized anxiety disorder, and obsessive-compulsive disorder; 48% did not feel comfortable in treating adult ADHD, but only 2% said they would refer for depression and 3% for generalized anxiety disorder. Only 34% thought they were very knowledgeable about adult ADHD.

Also, there is a good chance you may have other challenging health issues that have to be contended with, such as diabetes, hypertension, high cholesterol, and fibromyalgia-like pain disorders. If someone's primary care doctor doesn't feel comfortable managing ADHD, it does cause problems because many may not want to go to a "shrink" (psychiatrist), or their insurance coverage may make it more expensive.

Also, going to another doctor means more lost time from work. There also is no guarantee that the adult psychiatrist will make an accurate diagnosis leading to appropriate treatment. The take-home message is that if you strongly suspect you or a loved one have ADHD; you will likely have to search and specifically ask for a physician who does feel very knowledgeable in diagnosing and treating ADHD in adults.

- The medications to treat ADHD are schedule II drugs, so the physicians are worried it could lead to illicit use and possibly jeopardize their license.
- Physicians are concerned it could cause an addiction. This is rarely true unless the patient has a history of substance abuse issues. In contrast, many feel that treating ADHD could be an essential part of their recovery. Studies have demonstrated a 50% reduction in future substance abuse.
- Some think that medicating ADHD symptoms is tantamount to suppressing someone's uniqueness. Similarly, many used to think treating depression and bipolar disorder hamstring creativity.

David Woodman, MD et. al. recommended that all patients who present with significant mental health symptoms should be evaluated for ADHD because of the high prevalence rate in the general population and the high rate of comorbid psychiatric disorders (i.e., depression, anxiety, and substance use disorders). This is something I routinely do in my practice. There is progress in the mental health arena being made.

The clinic system I work in and others have recognized the importance of untreated depression and routinely screen for depression because of the significant impact on overall health. The greatest barrier was decreased confidence in diagnosing ADHD in addition to the stigma surrounding ADHD. Hopefully, with time, more doctors will routinely inquire about concentration, patience, and distractibility, just as they ask about vaccination, weight management, diet, smoking, and hypertension.

Dr. Joel Young, a psychiatrist from Michigan who wrote a chapter in his book on adolescent and adult ADHD entitled *ADHD, Fibromyalgia, chronic pain, and associated syndromes*, like me, observed that ADHD and other pain disorders occurred together frequently. He studied these relationships and will share his findings. His center is a referral center and has a large number of psychiatrists. Over 18 months, they evaluated patients who had ADHD and also reported having FM. Rheumatologists corroborated their diagnoses.

They discovered some enlightening observations. 70% had ADHD, and most were the inattentive type. Many of these patients reported pain reductions when they were prescribed stimulant medications. They looked at the effects of Vyvanse (LDX) on FM. Vyvanse is adderall with an amino acid attached that delays absorption allowing for a long acting adderall. The results were impressive with the FIQR (Fibromyalgia impact score) being cut in half.

They concluded that medications did not act directly as analgesics. Instead, they improved their ability to focus and function, aka TCB (taking care of business.) They were able to cope more effectively with their pain and fatigue.

Syndromes found to share higher rates of ADHD include:

- chronic fatigue syndrome
- irritable bowel
- tinnitus
- chronic headaches
- vulvodynia
- POTS, postural hypotension tachycardia syndrome

Most patients with these problems do not come in because of ADHD directly, but because of the physical manifestations of their regional pain problems. I share more about this in the chapter on the "faces of fibromyalgia." Many pursue medical treatment and often see the pain and rheumatology specialists who do not have any significant ADHD training. Treatments typically fall short, leading some to try alternative therapies or diagnoses like chronic Lyme disease. Most are left with marginal improvements, leading to incredible frustration.

The economic impact of lost wages or disability is very high. Many reading this book who have fibromyalgia, or who know someone who has, may currently be in the situation. There is hope to reverse the path you are on.

The fibro fog can be very challenging, but research points out that untreated ADHD is likely to play a significant role. Although infrequently assessed, diagnosis and subsequent treatment can be game changers. Treating ADHD can have impressive benefits for those with ADHD and chronic pain. Concentration, focus, and short-term memory are improved with the treatment of ADHD. Successful completion of tasks and improved ability to filter out pain to focus on tasks lead to a more optimistic mindset instead of a more pessimistic, catastrophizing outlook.

Chapter 8
Pediatrics and Fibromyalgia

1. Background
2. Colic
3. Restless Leg Syndrome
4. Abdominal migraines
5. Cyclical vomiting syndrome (CVS)
6. Postural orthostatic hypotension syndrome (POTS)
7. Juvenile Fibromyalgia

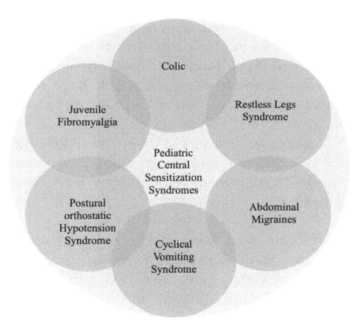

If you have fibromyalgia, there is a good chance that your problem started long before you were diagnosed. You likely had symptoms on the FM continuum going back to childhood, and possibly infancy. The most common childhood chronic pain disorders are growing pains, recurrent abdominal pain, and headaches in young children. By age 14, the most common pain disorders are headache, abdominal pain, and back pain.

Also, colic and POTS syndrome fall on the FM spectrum. If you have one pain disorder such as migraines, you have a higher chance of having other problems like irritable bowel syndrome. These childhood pain disorders are on the continuum with adult centralized pain disorders. For many women with fibromyalgia, their first problem was with painful menstrual periods, much worse than their 'girlfriends.' Often, absence from school was needed.

Similar underlying problems found in adults also make children have an increased underlying risk. One of those is stress. Like PTSD in adults, early-life adversity may increase risk in susceptible children to developing chronic pain disorders. Those who are more susceptible have ADHD, RLS, and familial history of chronic pain disorders. When measured at age 18-19, abuse in childhood was associated with a 97% increased risk of FM disorders in adulthood. The pain itself is a stressor and, as it evolves, may generate a positive feedback loop to increase anxiety levels and impact stress regulation.

Older adolescents who were born very prematurely (<26 weeks gestation) were more likely to report current pain of at least moderate severity, with increased pain intensity also associated with higher anxiety and pain catastrophizing scores. In adolescents, Chronic Widespread Pain was associated with anxiety, depression, conduct, and attentional problems. High self-esteem, seldom feeling lonely, family cohesion, and social confidence significantly buffer adolescents from developing FM like pain.

Colic

Did you know that colic can be considered the earliest pain disorder in children?

There is a connection between colic and chronic pain disorders. Infantile colic is a disease during the early months of life. It is also one of the most distressing challenges for parents. It is estimated that it affects 10% to 40% of the world's normal infant population. An infant with colic has bouts of inconsolable crying for more than 3 hours every day, more than three days every week, and longer than three weeks. It usually goes away by four months of age. In between these episodes, they are okay. The infant otherwise is growing and feeding well. Persistent crying throughout the day, fevers, poor feeding, and inadequate weight gain, however, should alert the parent and pediatrician that something more is going on.

Colic typically occurs late morning and evening to nighttime. Being held, rocked, and white noise exposure help lessen their distress. It can be very frustrating for a parent and the infant. When someone asks if you have a "good baby," colic is often the discriminating factor. If you are a parent with a colicky baby, you may not understand what is going on and feel inadequate or relatively helpless. It is associated with increased parental depression, disrupted breastfeeding, and even death in extreme cases due to exasperated parents hurting their babies by shaking them because they don't know what to do and are very frustrated.

I actively screen for colic at the 2-week visit. The next visit is not until two months old, so I alert parents to look for signs of colic. If colic develops, I like to take the time to educate you on what colic is. Just like in FM, education is the first step. For colic, understanding this mysterious and misunderstood problem, and that you aren't a bad parent is the start.

Research suggests that colic likely has to do with a sensitive, amplified central nervous system. For example, children who have migraines are about three times as likely to have had colic. Migraines are a disorder of central pain and pain augmentation. As with other central pain processing disorders besides colic, genetic predisposition appears to play a significant role. Usually, one of the parents has or had one of the fibromyalgia-like illnesses such as migraines, irritable bowel syndrome, or FM.

Medication treatment of colic has not been effective or safe with medications such as simethicone. Others, such as hyoscyamine, peppermint oil, and tea, have not been recommended due to safety or disruption of breastfeeding.

There appears to be a connection between dairy consumption by the infant either directly from cow milk protein-based formula or indirectly through the mother's intake of dairy. In one study, mothers who stopped drinking milk and eating dairy showed 13 of 19 had resolution of their colic, with 12 of the 13 having symptoms returning with reintroduction of cow's milk.

There also is a connection between colic and restless leg syndrome. One study showed infants who had colic had a 75% chance that one of the parents had restless leg syndrome (RLS). This strong connection should alert the pediatrician and the parent to be on the lookout for RLS symptoms as their child grows older. It is likely that the parent has not been officially diagnosed with RLS as most adults with it have just endured and normalized it. This is an opportunity to help the parent suffering with RLS to be identified and treated as well.

Restless Leg Syndrome (RLS)

The vast majority of pediatric RLS patients present to the doctor with the parental complaint of poor, restless sleep. Many parents will be given sleep hygiene advice, which, unfortunately, doesn't help significantly with RLS. Ineffective behavioral intervention, too, can lower a parent's parenting confidence. "What am I doing wrong? I do all the steps, and he or she still doesn't sleep well."

Small children, infants, and preschoolers with RLS may have difficulty initiating sleep, awakening frequently, and demanding the presence of caregivers to begin or return to sleep. Almost inconsolable crying is very common, and children are commonly brought to sleep for the rest of the night with their parents. Parents then note extreme stirring, with such frequent kicking and position changing that the parents' sleep is disturbed. Children with RLS frequently move their legs in bed while sleeping. In a very typical movement, infants may raise both legs and beat them vigorously against the mattress, or continuously rub their legs against each other. It is common to hear stories of patients whose friends, siblings, or cousins never wanted to sleep in the same bed with them during childhood sleepovers because they moved so much.

Restless legs syndrome (RLS), also known as Willis–Ekbom disease, is a common pediatric neurological condition affecting 2–4% of school-aged children and adolescents. Symptoms range from mild to severe with 25–50% of pediatric cases having moderate to severe symptoms. Both adult and pediatric RLS can adversely impact sleep, mood, cognition, and quality of life. The pathophysiology of RLS has been defined with genetics and the brain dopamine system playing big roles.

International Restless Legs Syndrome Study Group consensus diagnostic criteria for restless legs syndrome.

Restless legs syndrome (RLS), a neurological sensorimotor disorder often profoundly disturbing sleep, is diagnosed by ascertaining a syndrome that consists of all of the following features:

- An urge to move the legs usually but not always accompanied by or felt to be caused by uncomfortable and unpleasant sensations in the legs
- The urge to move the legs and any accompanying unpleasant sensations begin or worsen during periods of rest or inactivity such as lying down or sitting
- The urge to move the legs and any accompanying unpleasant sensations are partially or totally relieved by movement, such as walking or stretching, at least as long as the activity continues
- The urge to move the legs and any accompanying unpleasant sensations during rest or inactivity only occur or are worse in the evening or night than during the day
- The occurrence of the above features is not solely accounted for as symptoms primary to another medical or a behavioral condition (e.g., myalgia, venous stasis, leg edema, arthritis, leg cramps, positional discomfort, habitual foot tapping)

Medical professionals have developed criteria for diagnosing RLS in children ages 2 through 12 years with
1. Definite,
2. Probable or
3. Possible RLS

Definite RLS:
1. A child feels an urge to move the legs that begins or worsens with sitting or lying down.

2. Partially or totally relieved by movement. The urge is worse in the evening or night than during the day or occurs exclusively in the evening or nighttime hours.
3. Children describe the discomfort using their own words, such as "owies, tickle, tingle, static, bugs, spiders, ants, boo-boos, want to run, a lot of energy in my legs," etc.
4. There is a clinical sleep disturbance for age.
5. A biological parent or sibling has RLS. A sleep study has documented a periodic limb movement index of 5 or more per hour of sleep.

Probable RLS:
1. There is an urge to move the legs.
2. and the move begins or worsens with sitting or lying down.
3. The urge to move is partially or totally relieved by movement,
4. and the child has a biological parent or sibling with definite RLS.

Possible RLS:
1. The child has PLMD,
2. and a biological parent or sibling has definite RLS,
3. but the child does not meet the criteria for definite or probable childhood RLS.

Adolescents (13 years and older) are evaluated with the adult criteria.

Behavioral insomnia, also known as bad sleep habits like watching videos or playing video games in bed, is frequent in those with RLS. These are understandable because if you can't sleep and can't turn your mind off, you can at least distract yourself with stimulating videos or games. These are frequently present with the typical symptoms of chronic sleep deprivation, such as poor academic performance, irritability, daytime fatigue, and FM disorders. All patients diagnosed with childhood behavioral insomnia deserve screening for RLS, and if identified, treated appropriately.

Because of their poor sleep, children do not have an entirely healthy day. Younger children become agitated and sometimes even turbulent, and tantrum spells are frequent. They also do not appear fatigued. Instead, they behave restlessly. Older children have difficulty waking up in the morning. They manifest long periods of sleep inertia, difficulty getting out of bed in the morning. It is vital to discriminate RLS from irregular sleep schedules from school days to weekends that many children adopt. Fatigue is commonly stated by older RLS patients, mainly in the afternoon, and academic performance is often mediocre. ADHD is more common in RLS patients than in unaffected children.

Bad sleep habits are more likely to develop in those with RLS. Due to difficulty falling asleep, children are prone to delay going to bed. Conflicts among parents and children are frequent, as parents believe that their children are lazy, mainly concerning school duties. Treatment for children with RLS is the medications used in adults but at lower doses, which was discussed in the section on sleep.

These medications are considered off label as the now generic drug companies have not gone through the expensive studies to prove effectiveness and safety. Rarely in children, iron deficiency can be a cause. High levels of exercise can diminish and sometimes eliminate symptoms of RLS symptoms. This variability of activity is why RLS symptoms are less during the summer or a very active sport or dance season, for example.

Despite the high prevalence of RLS and the high percentage of RLS sufferers with symptoms that impact on activities of daily living, RLS remains underdiagnosed and also misdiagnosed-- as skin irritation, arthritis, malingering, and vein disorders in adults, and as growing pains.

Abdominal Migraines

Abdominal migraine is a form of migraine seen mainly in children. It is most common in children ages five to nine years old but can also occur in adults. It consists primarily of abdominal pain, nausea, and vomiting.

The primary symptom is abdominal pain. However, when patients are directly asked, they typically have some level of headache associated with the episodes. As they go through puberty, the abdominal pain diminishes and transforms into more of a typical migraine. They also are more likely to develop painful menstrual cramps than average. There also may be development of IBS as time goes on.

The pain associated with abdominal migraine is generally located in the middle of the abdomen around the belly button. It is often described as dull or "just sore" and may be moderate to severe. Along with the pain, there can be loss of appetite, nausea, vomiting, and pallor. The attacks last between 3-72 hours, and in between attacks, there should be complete symptom freedom.

Like other fibromyalgia-like pain disorders, several factors can build up where a tipping point is achieved, and the abdominal migraine symptoms spill over. In children, the most common factor is poor sleep. This includes inconsistent bedtimes and wake times. Irregular sleep schedules are commonly seen with different weekend bedtimes compared to school day bedtimes. A child might be going to bed at 8 PM, getting up at 6 AM during school days but on the weekends, and is allowed to stay up until 11 PM and get up at 8 AM.

The abdominal migraine is often delayed a couple of days after the change. It may not occur the Saturday after a Friday night sleepover. Instead, it may occur Monday during school or after school when they couldn't fall asleep until 11 PM on Sunday night and are forced to get up at 6 AM to get ready for school.

Stress can play a role, depending on the home environment. Increased anxiety and untreated ADHD may affect the response to stress as well. Worry may interfere with the ability to fall asleep. Many may suffer from untreated Restless Leg Syndrome as well. Consistent high levels of exercise can temper the symptoms. It is common to have the symptoms disappear during the summer when children have more opportunities to be much more physically active. However, when school starts, the transition from summer hours is replaced by having a lot more time being sedentary and getting up much earlier. The child may think that it is a reward or special privilege to stay up late.

Diet also can play a role. A diet high in processed carbs, meats, dairy, and oils seems to increase risk, whereas a diet higher in fruits, vegetables, whole grains, and minimally added oils and fats have a protective effect. Read more on nutrition in the chapter on the treatment of FM.

If a child does have ADHD, their anxiety level may be higher. If they have the drive to succeed in school, they may need to spend more time after school doing homework and exercise less. They may substitute video games, TV, and other electronic media in place of the exercise that their body needs to function the best.

Medications like Tylenol, NSAIDs, and triptans can be effective. Still, prevention by a healthy lifestyle can go a long way to prevent them. If underlying Restless Leg Syndrome is present, treatment is essential. RLS, as previously discussed, can sometimes be treated if exercise can hit a high level. Rarely iron deficiency can contribute, but most often, this is a genetic problem, and medication is needed.

Most would start with gabapentin, ropinirole, or pramipexole. These medications are effective in treating children with RLS but have only been FDA approved for the treatment of RLS in adults, like many other medicines. There are studies demonstrating the safe use of these for RLS and pain conditions as young as premature infants.

Cyclical Vomiting Syndrome

In 1998, during residency, I presented the case of the week, the most interesting and educational case to the senior doctors, residents, and medical students. I had a mysterious 15-year-old patient who had experienced recurrent episodes of severe vomiting and was admitted to the hospital on a couple of occasions. He was missing over 1/3 of his classes from being ill. He seemed to be avoiding school.

These were happening once a month and lasted a few days. He had headaches associated with them, along with light and sound sensitivity. He had multiple tests done, which all were normal. He was missing more and more school. It seemed to many caring for him that he could be malingering or faking it. He had worsened over time and avoided school so often that his mom had decided to home school him.

What was this mysterious illness?

He had cyclical vomiting syndrome. This disorder predominantly occurs in children. Cyclical vomiting syndrome (CVS) is characterized by discrete episodes of recurrent, profuse vomiting. These are resolved within a discrete time and with periods of well-being between the attacks. Each episode is often stereotypical for the individual in terms of onset, duration, and symptoms but may vary between individuals. The vomiting can be profuse and associated with extreme nausea and lethargy.

Each attack can be debilitating as the child sometimes spends days being hospitalized for intravenous hydration. CVS classically has four phases: inter-episodic, prodromal, vomiting, and recovery. The time in between they feel fairly well. The prodrome is the time before the vomiting begins, often a couple of hours when one feels fatigued, tired, run-down, and may yawn more often. The vomiting occurs and then recovery when the fatigue, residual nausea, and light and sound sensitivity gradually fade.

There is a link between CVS and migraine, suggestive of a central nervous system etiology. Both conditions have symptoms of nausea, photophobia, and headache and have similar triggers of stress and sleep. Migraine headaches do not typically have vomiting but sometimes do. Those with CVS often have headaches. Both last a similar duration of 3-72 hours. Interestingly, there is often a co-existing personal or family history of migraines in individuals with CVS.

Also, many patients may spend months of repeated hospital admissions before a diagnosis is made. Patients are often misdiagnosed as food poisoning, gastroesophageal reflux disease, or peptic ulcer disease.

The diagnosis of CVS remains primarily one of exclusion. In a child with recurrent vomiting, it is essential to rule out life-threatening conditions such as gastrointestinal structural anomalies, including malrotation with volvulus, brain tumors, and inborn errors in metabolism. Children with epilepsy can occasionally present with recurrent vomiting, especially if it involves the occipital lobe. For fibromyalgia and other central pain disorders, filtering through the possible causes consists of taking a careful history, physical exam, and appropriate testing, which can rule these out. Treatment during the vomiting includes IV fluids, nausea medicine, and a calm dark environment.

Prevention includes improving sleep, which includes good sleep hygiene, similar to migraines. Consistent bedtime and wake time are especially important. In migraine patients, restless leg syndrome (RLS) as a comorbid disorder seems to be increased, ranging from 9% to 39%. It is crucial to assess for underlying RLS and, if present, treat. Amitriptyline is a medication shown to be effective with CVS as well. It works by increasing serotonin and norepinephrine levels, which are lower in those with FM disorders, and improves sleep. Diet appears to play a role, similar to irritable syndrome. Limiting dairy, meat, and caffeine is helpful. Having a diet high in fruits, vegetables, beans and lentils, and whole grains is beneficial.

Children and adolescents with cyclic vomiting syndrome are more likely to have psychiatric disorders, especially anxiety disorders. Studies are limited in CVS, but migraine studies show the increased presence of ADHD. A study demonstrated that there was a four times greater risk of having ADHD in those with migraines. The risk increased to 7 times higher in those with the most severe migraines. CVS could be classified as severe on the migraine spectrum. Clinical experience strongly supports that the treatment of ADHD can reduce migraines. Untreated ADHD may explain episodes of increased stress, inducing the CVS episodes. For example, the school project or exam every couple weeks may crescendo in a last-minute frenzy of stress the presence of CVS should prompt screening for ADHD.

Postural Orthostatic Hypotension Syndrome (POTS)

POTS is a chronic multisystem disorder involving a broader array of symptoms than the orthostatic tachycardia that defines it. Many patients are diagnosed with comorbidities along with POTS. Like fibromyalgia, most people with POTS have seen multiple physicians before the diagnosis, which is most often made by cardiologists as opposed to rheumatologists, as is common with FM. This higher rate of diagnosis by cardiologists is likely because the most common symptoms include lightheadedness, fast heart rate, and near fainting episodes.

Postural orthostatic tachycardia syndrome (POTS) occurs commonly during adolescence, with the most common age of onset being 14 and shares many of the features of central pain syndromes like migraines, CFS, and fibromyalgia. It happens much more often in young women, manifesting with symptoms of fatigue, headaches, palpitations, sleep disturbance, nausea, and bloating. There are many opinions on the causes, but it appears to have, similar to fibromyalgia, multiple factors involved.

Is POTS another face of fibromyalgia-like pain syndromes?

This syndrome is relatively new and was first described in 1999. The predominant viewpoint initially was dysregulation of heart rate control. During a tilt table test, the heart races very fast, and blood pressure drops. Much initial attention has been focused on this as a cardiovascular problem. Still, new research has found that most diagnosed people do not meet the blood pressure and heart rate criteria, and many with chronic fatigue and sedentary people do. Half of the patients with POTS have never fainted, and 30% have about once a year. Also, the tilt table test doesn't consistently help discriminate POTS from other pain disorders.

Besides symptoms of lightheadedness with standing, many POTS patients report incapacitating cognitive dysfunction or "brain fog" even while lying down or seated. Studies comparing POTS with chronic fatigue syndrome (CFS) show similar fatigue, daytime sleepiness, anxiety, and depression. 75% of those with POTS and 80% of those with CFS and POTS reported wanting to exercise but feel they can't. Many in both report that a preceding infection caused the illnesses among other causes as well, although research suggests this is more likely an association and not a causation.

POTS patients have higher subjective daytime sleepiness, fatigue, worse sleep, and appear to play a factor in about 50% of their health-related quality of life. Studies show a big difference in the subjective time it takes to fall and stay asleep. They have a decreased sense of feeling refreshed with awakening compared to healthy controls.

Adolescents with postural tachycardia syndrome (POTS) often experience ill-defined cognitive impairment referred to by patients as "brain fog." The top-ranked descriptors of brain fog by patients are "forgetful," "cloudy," and "difficulty focusing, thinking, and communicating." The most frequently reported brain-fog triggers were fatigue (91%), lack of sleep (90%), lightheadedness with prolonged standing (87%), dehydration (86%), and feeling faint (85%). 86% reported impairment in school-related activities.

Below are the most common descriptors by percentage that patients with POTS used when asked to describe the brain fog they experience:

- forgetful 91%,
- difficulty thinking 89%,
- difficulty focusing 88%,
- cloudy 88%,
- trouble finding the right words/communicating 88%,
- mental fatigue 86%,
- slow 86%,
- mind went blank 85%,
- spacey 83%,
- difficulty processing what others say 80%,
- exhausted 80%,
- easily distracted 77%,
- difficulty processing words read 75%,
- thoughts moving too quickly 40%

These symptoms probably sound familiar to you. These are the same difficulties those with ADHD and CFS (Chronic fatigue Syndrome) report. In the same study, 67% of the patients treated with the stimulants used for ADHD reported improvement in "brain fog" symptoms. Other studies have shown that those with POTS have the ADHD inattentive and not the hyperactive subtype. The primary abnormality noted in patients with POTS was difficulty with maintaining attention.

ADHD also is noticed less in childhood compared to adolescence. This discrepancy may reflect that girls tend to be less noticed for their ADHD symptoms than boys who are more likely to have hyperactive symptoms than girls who are more often inattentive. The delay in recognition may indicate a higher IQ in those with POTS, which may buffer them from being diagnosed earlier.

Along with ADHD, differences in anxiety in those with POTS were found using the Beck anxiety index (BAI) but not the anxiety symptom index (ASI). The BAI showed a moderately high level in those with POTS. A major difference between the BAI and ASI is that the BAI measures both somatic (body) pain and subjective anxiety and panic symptoms. In contrast, the ASI measures sensitivity to anxiety-provoking stimuli but not body pain symptoms. This finding is consistent with fibromyalgia-like pain, where there are higher rates of ADHD and anxiety.

Forty percent of people with POTS have a history of migraines, with 94% reporting problems with headaches. Only 30% have been diagnosed with irritable bowel syndrome (IBS), yet 90% have nausea, 83% with abdominal pain, 79% with bloating, 71% with constipation, and 69% with diarrhea. Only 20% of patients were diagnosed with fibromyalgia, yet 84% reported muscle pains. These findings suggest that fibromyalgia pain syndromes like functional dyspepsia, IBS, and fibromyalgia in those with POTS are underdiagnosed and underrecognized. These findings also suggest a common central pain disorder problem as with other fibromyalgia-like pain disorders.

Treatment of POTS

The approach for treatment is similar to other central pain/fibromyalgia-like diseases. More will be discussed in the chapter on treatment. Exercise plays an important role but has to be done differently than those rehabbing from other injuries who do not have fibromyalgia-like disorders. There tends to be significant deconditioning in those with POTS. Start at a low level and gradually increase the exercise.

A friend of mine wanted to run a marathon but had been relatively sedentary. He didn't try to join a friend who was already running marathons. If he would, he would be extremely sore and unable to continue. Similar to those with POTS, higher intensity or amount of exercise from baseline can be more distressing.

Instead of high intensity and duration of exercise, he started with a reasonable goal of something he knew he could achieve. He walked for 20 minutes every day. He added 5 minutes each week until he got to 30 minutes. He would then add a little jogging during the 30 minutes of walking before moving over weeks to jog the 30 minutes. Each subsequent week, he added another 5 minutes of jogging. With time he was able to build to the point where he ran his 26-mile marathon. A similar approach should be used with POTS, "start low, and go slow." Studies have found a regular cardiovascular exercise program to have profound physiological and clinical benefits in POTS patients. In addition, eating a healthy diet is essential.

It is also important to be assessed for ADHD and restless leg syndrome, and if present to treat. Studies for POTS and CFS demonstrated significant improvement in those treated with psychostimulants. Also, the treatment of RLS when present, as well as good sleep hygiene, is beneficial.

Juvenile Fibromyalgia

Juvenile fibromyalgia (JFM), a chronic disorder of widespread musculoskeletal pain in combination with autonomic, sensory, and cognitive dysfunction, is responsible for considerable morbidity and impaired quality of life in affected patients and their families. Historically, fibromyalgia has been incorrectly characterized as a psychosomatic or psychogenic disorder, but new understanding of the science of pain has demonstrated unambiguously that it is an organic disorder of the pain processing system itself.

JFM is characterized by widespread pain, sleep difficulty, fatigue and numerous other associated symptoms. Several studies have documented high levels of physical, emotional and social impairment in adolescent JFM patients that persist over time. Current treatment approaches for JFM include medications to manage pain and improve sleep, and recommendations for physical activity and aerobic exercise and/or cognitive-behavioral therapy to improve daily functioning and coping.

As with other pain syndromes centralized pain where there is no identifiable nerve or tissue damage. It is the result of persistent neuronal dysregulation involving overactive ascending pain pathways, and a deficiency of descending inhibitory pain pathways. The prevalence of children is about 3-6% in 10- to 19-year-olds. The same kinds of symptoms found in adults are also found in children. Generalized aches and pains are universal, along with headache and sleep disturbances in the majority.

Criteria for diagnosing juvenile fibromyalgia have been developed.

Major Criteria
- *Generalized musculoskeletal pain at three or more sites for three or more months*
- *No underlying medical condition*
- *Normal laboratory tests*
- *Five or more typical tender points*
- *Minor Criteria- Presence of three of the following features:*
- *Chronic anxiety or tension*
- *Fatigue*

- *Poor sleep*
- *Chronic headache*
- *Irritable bowel syndrome*
- *Subjective soft tissue swelling*
- *Numbness*
- *Pain modulation by physical activities*
- *Pain modulation by weather factors*
- *Pain modulation by anxiety or stress*

Tender points in adults are not required for the diagnosis of FM. Assessment of tender points is subjective and open to interpretation. I do not feel it is needed for diagnosis. The adult criteria have not excluded FM diagnosis if they have another underlying medical disease like rheumatoid arthritis. About half of adults with RA have fibromyalgia.

Early detection of JFM is an indication of a better prognosis, with significant gains in quality of life, and functionality for individuals who receive adequate treatment, whereas those with widespread pain that are not treated adequately have a greater chance of developing fibromyalgia. On the other hand, in a large prospective longitudinal study of JFM patients found that the majority of adolescent patients (~80%) with JFM seen in a pediatric specialty care setting continued to report persistent pain and other FM symptoms as they transitioned into young adulthood.

Key Take-home Points:

- **Guidelines agree that the diagnosis remains clinical, and the purpose of the physical examination and limited laboratory investigations is to rule out some other somatic disease that can sufficiently explain the symptoms.**

you seek medical attention. One example is someone who has chronic fatigue, who later develops chest pain with exertion instead of a decrease in intensity. This exertional chest pain is in contrast to the expected reduction during exercise with fibromyalgia. Another example would be developing unexpected weight loss and bloody stools, which could be a sign of inflammatory bowel disease or cancer instead of irritable bowel syndrome.

2. **There is typically no one magic pill.**
    Treatment involves multiple approaches starting with education, certain medications, optimization of exercise and sleep, a whole-foods plant-based diet, and counseling to help guide you on effective coping strategies. By now, I hope you have received an excellent education on what fibromyalgia is and don't feel labeled as having FM by a doctor because "she couldn't find anything else wrong with me." Understanding the role you play in getting healthy is essential. Using baseball terminology, this is a game of more singles than home runs. Each intervention is unlikely to hit a home run. On average, you can expect about 25% to 50% improvement with each intervention, but the results will vary individually and to the extent of implementation. You also will be facing obstacles that can increase fibromyalgia symptoms and hijack good intentions. It is like a tug of war.

Fibromyalgia Management

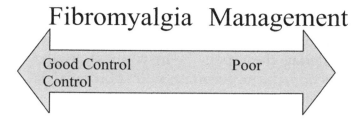

Good Control   Poor
Control

A plant-based diet
Consistent exercise
Good sleep
Appropriate Medications

Poor Diet
(Low Fiber high in
processed carbs,
added fats, and
animal protein)
Inconsistent exercise
Poor Sleep Hygiene

Treated ADHD
Treated RLS
Low Stress
(good management of
stress)

Untreated ADHD
Untreated RLS
High stress
Stopping appropriate
medications
PMS

3. **It is crucial to have patience. Your chronic pain likely** hasn't started overnight, and, by now, you hopefully have a deeper understanding of fibromyalgia. Each intervention in the process will work in concert with the others. We will talk about the roles of exercise, diet, and medications. When you look back at times when you have had the least amount of FM symptoms, you are likely to recall times when you were the most regularly active and sleeping well and had the least amount of stress. There may have been a gradual change or sudden change that has gotten you to the

point where you are now. Now, look to rebuild back to where you were before with a comprehensive approach.

4. **Reconsider your expectations. It is going to take more than medications to feel and function the best.**

I will discuss the role of exercise, diet, sleep, appropriate diagnoses, and tailored medication approaches that impact your healing. We have many treatments for medical problems where you are a very passive receiver. Most infectious diseases are treated simply by receiving an antibiotic. All you have to do is open the pill bottle, take a pill with a swallow of water, wait for the medication to get absorbed into the bloodstream, go to the site of infection and work with the immune system to kill the bacteria. There is no stigma from your family or friends for taking the antibiotic, but there might be if you make significant diet changes by eating a whole-foods plant-based to treat your fibromyalgia.

5. **If you have a doctor who says they don't believe in fibromyalgia, consider getting a second opinion.**

FM is real, even if your doctor doesn't think so. You are working with your doctor as an ally as you navigate this challenging and initially overwhelming syndrome. A doctor who says they don't believe in it is not going to be effective in helping you. Most doctors want to help you, but don't know their blind spot. This book may be helpful for your physician.

Fibromyalgia is a blind spot.

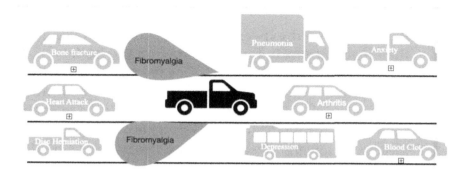

6. **Sleep is Key.**

    Patients who recover from FM fall asleep quickly, sleep deeply and wake up refreshed. If you are sleeping deeply, the autonomic nervous system is in a relaxed mood. You feel safe. You wake up refreshed. Good sleep can be easier said than done for various reasons, and there may be medical problems, not just bad sleep habits or stress to overcome. We will dig into this further.

7. **Monitor your symptoms, life, and self-care.**

    Make feeling better your priority. This starts with carefully tracking your life. What does this mean? A simple journal like the outline that I have at the end of the section will build awareness and through awareness empowerment. Lifestyle decisions you make do have a very important impact on how you feel living with fibromyalgia. You don't know what your average number of steps a day currently are. You may not realize you are only getting 2,000 steps a day on average and how much your activity varies within the day and from day to day. You will learn more about exercise in the next chapter.

Planning is very important in managing your FM. Like many with FM, you are not the best at planning. This may be related to untreated ADHD. Like a student who has daily assignments and a homework and project checklist, the fibromyalgia checklist acts in a similar way as a reminder of important things that you need to focus on.

A big semester project a student has is best done if it is paced out on a daily basis. This is similar to managing FM.

Chapter 10
Exercise

If you are like many people living with fibromyalgia, you currently are not very active and may be the least active you have ever been in your life. Studies monitoring activity level in FM revealed low engagement in moderate-vigorous activity with over 95% of patients not meeting recommended guidelines of physical activity. Each of you reading this with FM or who have a loved one with FM are at different levels of activity on the spectrum. Some may be only doing activities of daily living struggling to get even 1,000 steps in a day. Others may be getting 10,000 steps but still struggling.

What do you very likely have in common with most other people who have fibromyalgia but probably don't realize?

Earlier in your life, you likely used to be very active compared to your current levels.

You as a child may have played sports, danced, or road bikes, but likely kept very busy in some way. Maybe you worked a lot. You may have been one of the coaches' favorite players because you were the first to practice and the last to leave. Your drive to be active might have been because you would have preferred exercise than to do homework. A patient, 20 years old, recently diagnosed with IBS, RLS and ADHD used to care for horses in middle school and most of high school. She would work 4 hrs. after school and up to 8 hours a day on the weekend and during the summer.

Now in college she worked part time as a waitress and worked out twice a week for an hour at the fitness center. This reduction in exercise wasn't something done intentionally to cause her IBS to flare up. She also had been completely unaware how her work caring for horses was treating her IBS, RLS and ADHD. Not until college did the symptoms crescendo when her activity plummeted.

You have a memory of what it was like to be active and felt good doing it. Who would have imagined back then that you would develop fibromyalgia's struggles in the future? If this is you, I want you to know that you are not alone, and there is a path back.

How did you get to your current situation?

One pattern seen with FM is progression and increased diagnoses as people get older. Prevalence of FM rises in middle age, and peaks at 7.4% among those 70 to 79 years old. The increase in prevalence is also seen in other chronic pain disorders. As we discussed earlier, activity levels on the average drop as people get older. Compared with age-matched control patients, women with fibromyalgia are less physically active as measured with step counters, have significantly lower perceived functional ability, and demonstrate impaired physical performance. Several exercise studies have shown that persons with fibromyalgia can engage in moderate and even vigorous exercise; however, in many studies, participants experienced difficulties performing and adhering to strenuous and even moderate-intensity regimens because of increased fibromyalgia symptoms.

For people who are susceptible to FM or have FM they need to be regularly much more active than those who don't have FM. On the continuum of FM susceptibility those who are unaffected could be sedentary for a week and feel the same as if they would have been walking 10,000-20,000 steps a day. However, if you have FM and you don't exercise for a week, you are likely to feel a lot more pain. It is like water skiing. To hydroplane on the water one with FM would need a higher speed than one without to stay above the water.

Aerobic exercise has been demonstrated to be effective at improving outcomes for a wide range of chronic medical conditions. Reviews of the exercise literature suggest that in FM, aerobic exercise programs improve overall symptoms and pain. In an especially well-conducted study involving a 20-week supervised cardiovascular fitness training program, 18 FM patients demonstrated significant improvement in cardiovascular fitness scores and clinically meaningful improvements in pain threshold scores.

A second study showed a short-term benefit of aerobic exercise in FM patients compared to a group that received stress management. The reason for the beneficial effect of exercise on symptoms in these conditions is likely multifactorial. Aerobic exercise may influence endogenous analgesic systems while also increasing a sense of well-being and control.

A study using medical imaging confirmed that increased physical activity has a positive effect on pain perception in women with fibromyalgia. It demonstrated that higher levels of self-reported and accelerometer-monitored physical activity in women with fibromyalgia were associated with decreases in pain ratings and "greater responses in pain regulatory brain regions while receiving painful stimuli."

A study from the University of Wisconsin compared those with FM to those without and fMRI changes in the brain and response to the impact of exercise on pain. The fMRIs demonstrated the brain response to exercise in the areas involved in pain control. The effect of training on the central nervous system involvement in pain modulation as well as mechanisms underlying the pain-relieving effects of exercise in FM demonstrated that a relatively short bout of cycling (25 minutes) exercise resulted in improvements in pain modulation in FM. Study results suggest that exercise appeared to stimulate brain regions involved in descending pain inhibition in FM patients, decreasing their sensitivity to pain. Thus, exercise may benefit patients with FM via improving the functional capacity of the pain modulatory system. Think of it as the guitar amplifier that has had its volume turned down.

Key Point: Exercise turns down the pain amplifier.

So great, now what? The more I exercise, the more I hurt. How can exercise be good for me? This sentiment is common, and the dilemma deserves a remedy. You probably know exercise is good but have unknowingly done some things that have sabotaged your efforts. We will dig into that further.

What exercise should I do?

There are many options but consider something you enjoy. Your current level of exercise and underlying mechanical problems like significant arthritis also play an important role. Each person reading this is in their own unique situation with its unique challenges. You may be 65-years old, weigh 450 lbs., have significant arthritis in your knee and hip joints along with diffuse body pain. Or you may be 16 years old with no arthritis at all but be severely deconditioned. The choices and options will be different for each person. For the more severely affected by arthritis you will be "differently-abled." You might have significant spinal stenosis, making walking with a normal gait challenging, but using a walker, biking with a recumbent bike, and doing modified yoga or pilates may be necessary.

Consider low-impact exercises such as walking, swimming, or stationary cycling to reduce the pain associated with exercise. Investigators have found a gradual progression in exercise intensity and a focus on the most effective adherence to a lifelong program. Look at this with the long term in mind. One of the challenges with exercise is adherence. This has been demonstrated in many studies with a higher dropout rate in the exercise group.

How do I exercise?

For many, exercise has been an uncomfortable word, similar to taking a bad-tasting medicine. I recommend getting an activity monitor and wearing it for a week. The first week gives you a baseline for your activity. You will likely observe with this self-experiment that you have a maladaptive behavior most others with fibromyalgia unconsciously do as well. This bad habit is that your levels of exercise vary like a roller coaster. Notice the differences of a typical FM patient vs one who is managing it more effectively.

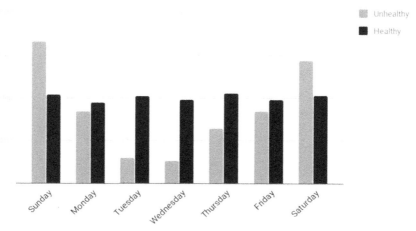

Steps per day in Unhealthy vs Healthy activity in FM patients

Typically, you may rest for a couple of days after feeling bad and then do 2-4 times more than your baseline for a day or two and then feel wiped out and are at higher levels of pain. You then rest a couple of days until you feel better and then repeat the cycle. Flattening the roller coaster to consistent, steady levels can improve FM symptoms by about 30%. The flattening results are similar to what we can expect from medication, and there are no side effects.

If your exercise at baseline ranges from 1000 to 5000 steps a day, it is essential to try to average 3000 steps a day for the first week. It would even be better to spread those steps out over a 16-hr. daytime than to do them all at once. Putting this to practice might involve getting up every hour and walking 200 steps, which over 16 hours = 3200 steps in a day. Each week gradually increase your daily step count by 10%. This process is known as pacing, and it also helps prevent an overuse injury such as tendonitis or plantar fasciitis, which could lead to a setback.

Week 2= 3500 steps
Week 3= 3900 steps
Week 4= 4300 steps
Week 5= 4700 steps
Week 6= 5200 steps
Week 7= 5700 steps
Week 8= 6300 steps
Week 9= 6900 steps
Week 10= 7600 steps
Week 11= 8400 steps
Week 12= 9200 steps
Week 13= 10,100 steps

Average number of daily steps

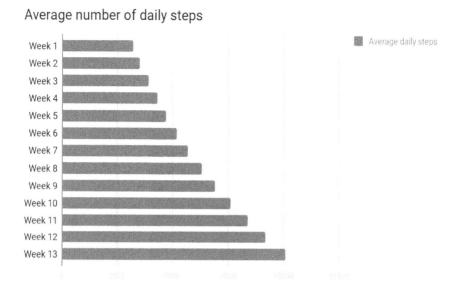

In about three months, you have increased your steps to over 10,000 steps. From my experience, most with FM require 10,000+ steps a day to feel the best. Once you are at that level, be consistent, and do your best to avoid significant changes. If walking is a challenge, then biking or swimming or chair exercises are alternatives as well.

Just as pacing activity during the week, daily activity level is optimally spread out over the whole day instead of consolidated in high levels during short time periods with being relatively sedentary the rest of the day. Many careers naturally are very active throughout the day. A nurse or carpenter naturally is active throughout the day. The graph below demonstrates an example of optimal vs suboptimal activity levels as measured by hourly step count during the day. Pacing throughout the day is ideal. This is why many who had careers that naturally paced them throughout the day struggle unknowingly when they retire.

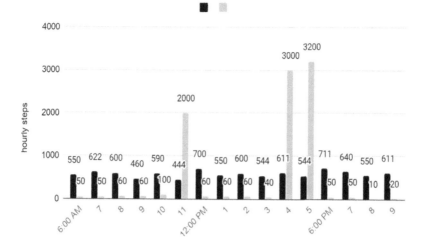

Pacing: Optimal vs Suboptimal hourly steps

It may be surprising, but most who have fibromyalgia were very active earlier in life before they developed fibromyalgia type symptoms. Many may have been athletes, but, if not into sports, played a lot as children, busy working on the farm, or in dance. Interestingly, as life circumstances change and you grow older, exercise levels often decrease, and the FM symptoms increase.

If you have fibromyalgia, the best memories retrospectively were your most regularly physically active, had the least stress, and were sleeping the best. It is not uncommon living here in Wisconsin with the Midwest's cold winters to have fibromyalgia peak from November through March and lessen through the summer. Outdoor yard work and exercise is diminished and not replaced with indoor training during the colder months with shorter amounts of daylight. This downward spiral can lead to worsening pain, sleep, and fibro fog leading to less exercise.

Key point: Just knowing that exercise is essential is a great start.

A patient of mine, "Rachel," had been doing great in the summer averaging 20,000 steps a day, but her fibro flared to a high level by the time she saw me in February. Her steps had dropped to about 7,000 steps a day, which is still a moderate number of steps for someone who doesn't have fibro, but for her, it wasn't what she needed to feel her best. Her brain was sensitive and tended to "idle at a very high level when left in neutral." She required higher levels of exercise to activate the pain inhibition activity in her brain. Unfortunately, she didn't have this insight and was somewhat reactive to the climate without corresponding compensation as the weather changed.

Rachel had small children she took to the park during the summer, did house and yard work, and ran for an hour in the evening. Around November, the yard work was no longer needed; it felt too cold to take the kids to the park, and with school starting, she had gotten out of the routine of going to the fitness center to run on the treadmill. Being aware of this is motivating to make keeping activity a priority, just like taking medication.

I have had more than one patient, though, that had this insight before becoming their doctor. When asked about their exercise, they might say, *"Dr. Lenz, I need to exercise vigorously daily for my mental health, to feel normal."*

If this resonates with you or with someone you love, then put the exercise into a plan. Write out daily goals and track them. If your loved one is going through this, try gentleness and respect and encourage them to increase their activity level gradually. Be patient as well. You may notice some soreness at times as you increase exercise levels, which is normal. As you build momentum, you will start to see changes. Sometimes this isn't apparent as it happens gradually. Using the FIQR score is very helpful and can reveal the effects of interventions over time.

Other exercises that may be helpful include yoga, pilates, Tai Chi, and strength training. For each of these, remember to start low and go slow. You will activate muscle groups you are not accustomed to using.

One final thought on exercise. Living with fibromyalgia can be like trying to water ski. You start in the water and have to be pulled up out of the water and then the speed and power has to be sufficient enough to keep you going. The inertia of getting out of the water can require a lot of strength and encouragement. If you are heavier or have weak upper body strength it can be a real challenge to get out of the water. Once you get on top of the water you plane out and are able to amazingly fly across the water. There is a minimum speed needed to stay on top of the water. When the speed starts to dip at and below the minimum threshold you start to sink and can get pulled back under the water. Similarly living with fibromyalgia is a lot like skiing. If your fibromyalgia impact score is very high, it can be very hard to even get out of the water.

Chapter 11
The Food Prescription

What if food could have a powerful effect on your fibromyalgia?

We eat every day and many times. Most people don't even think much about what they eat, let alone the powerful impact it has on the level of pain. You might be surprised by the significant impact that your diet can have on your health. Studies and many individual cases of success have demonstrated that a whole-foods plant-based (WFPB) diet can be a game changer.

There are many different diets, but the best way of eating is one of predominantly whole-plant foods. In addition to helping fibromyalgia and related disorders it has many other profound health benefits.

- Lower BMI (Body Mass Index), body fat
- Lower overall mortality
- Lower risk of ischemic heart disease
- Reduced Medication requirements
- Sustainable weight management
- Reduced high blood pressure, high cholesterol and high blood sugar
- Reduced risk of certain cancers, especially colorectal cancer
- Reduced inflammatory markers
- Reversal of advanced coronary artery disease
- Reversal of Type 2 Diabetes

In addition to all of these it will help with pain as well. I wanted to tell you about the effects of exercise and diet before medications. It is easy to take pills, but the effects of a healthy lifestyle are in my opinion even more important.

No doubt, losing weight can have profound reductions in suffering from conditions like hip and knee arthritis. Every extra pound you carry is felt to be 4 lbs. across your knee. If you are 100 or more lbs. over your healthy weight, your knees would feel like you lost 400+lbs. The last chapter just reviewed the benefits of exercise, but unfortunately exercise doesn't play a big role for weight loss. You can walk for an hour and burn off 600 Calories but then consume 600 Calories of calorie dense nutritionally depleted foods within minutes.

The vast majority of weight loss is related to the food you eat and not the portions. Eating a whole foods plant-based (WFPB) diet is the gold standard for a healthy diet for so many other health conditions including fibromyalgia and fibromyalgia-like pain syndromes. The same diet for reversing heart disease, diabetes, hypertension, and autoimmune diseases also reverses fibromyalgia and related disorders.

A study in 2001 using a raw, low-fat vegan diet showed an impressive reduction in fibromyalgia symptoms. The fibromyalgia impact questionnaire (FIQ) score dropped from an initial average of 51, which is in the moderate range to 37 after three months and 27 after 6 months of the diet change. The FIQ-R is used to measure the impact of fibromyalgia on life. A score in the 50s is moderately high, and in the 20s is a mildly elevated range.

All the parameters measured, including physical impairment, "feel good," pain, fatigue, rest, stiffness, anxiety, and depression, were reduced by about 50%. Initially only 15% of the subjects had scores <35. After 7 months 70% had scores < 35. This is more impressive than the results most have with medications. This study resulted in a 46% reduction in overall

FIQ score. A bigger decrease than seen by most people using a single medication.

In 2017, the first randomized controlled trial to examine the effects of a WFPB diet on subjective pain reports and functional status/ limitation due to fibromyalgia. The study found that a WFPB diet significantly improves various self-assessed measures of functional status among fibromyalgia patients.

A common misconception is that the use of a plant-based diet without animal products would lead to malnutrition. Except for a very small risk of B12 deficiency in those who commit 100% to the diet, a WFPB diet based on unrefined plant foods supplies the adequate amounts of calories, protein, fats, vitamins, and minerals including calcium, zinc, and iron. Interestingly, although the plant based dietary profile (low-fat, high fiber) can lead to a diet that is less energy dense and reduced caloric intake, the WFPB diet is associated with increased nutrient density as well as increased concentrations of several vitamins and trace minerals.

Other research suggests diet can have an impact on central pain-related diseases, including migraines, irritable bowel syndrome, and fibromyalgia. A study by Neal Barnard, MD showed a significant reduction in migraine frequency and intensity when going to a low fat WFPB diet. Pain improved with 87% reported they were "better" after the diet period, while only 50% in the omnivorous general diet felt better.

A WFPB diet is one with minimal added fat and includes whole grains, legumes, vegetables, fruits, nuts, seeds, and spices. Studies on a whole-foods plant-based diet have shown decreases in fatigue, which is often challenging to treat. There are different pathways on how this may improve symptoms. There is a strongly suspected role of the bacteria in the intestines, known as the microbiome, that strongly affect fibromyalgia symptoms. Several pathways are involved, one of which is short-chain fatty acids (SCFAs). They are two, three, and four carbon atom molecules formed when healthy bacteria in the intestines digest fiber. The three main types are acetate, propionate, and butyrate. These molecules are designed to work in concert with our bodies to keep us healthy in many ways. Each type of the many thousands of fibers we consume eating a whole-foods plant-based, fire up the production of SCFAs from the metabolic factories in the good gut bacteria.

One quick clarification. The fiber you eat is not your grandma's fiber; the Metamucil manufactured type taken in a slurry to help treat constipation. This form has limited benefits compared to the abundance of forms created in the vast diversity of plant fibers in whole-plant foods that have not been processed and stripped.

Many of you have heard of probiotics, which are colonies of healthy bacteria. The research shows mixed results on the benefits of probiotics by themselves. The mixed benefit is because they are similar to seeds that need good soil to grow in. That is where the prebiotics come in. Prebiotics are the healthy fibers that allow the good bacteria to thrive. Then there is a concept you likely are not familiar with, which is postbiotics. These are the compounds manufactured by the gut microbes when they get the raw material, fiber.

Prebiotics = Food for healthy gut bacteria
Probiotics = Microbes with good qualities
Postbiotics = Healthy compounds produced by gut microbes
On a simple level: Prebiotics + Probiotics = Postbiotics

Treatment with fiber fuels the good gut bacteria by activating them into vigorous, powerful, and consistent protectors and enhancers of health from the slumped over, rusty, and underutilized intestinal factories. Because they are acids, they increase the acidity of the intestines. In fact, there is a ten-fold higher level of acid production on a whole-foods plant-based diet. This acid changes the intestines' local ecosystem, suppressing the growth of dangerous strains like E Coli and Salmonella.

The more fiber consumed, the more effective the intestinal microbiome becomes in producing the SCFAs. This efficiency can be thought of as similar to muscle memory in athletic training or playing a musical instrument. The fiber also fuels the growth of beneficial bacterial colonies. This lack of healthy bacterial colonies to digest a large amount of fiber helps explain why one day of an exclusively WFPBD can cause discomfort. The gut has not been "trained" to handle that concentration of fiber. Similarly, someone who has been training for a marathon may easily knock off a 9-mile run on a Saturday, but their friend who only walks a mile 3 times a week struggles when he joins his friend on the 9-mile Saturday run. You have to train, but more on that later.

I have found myself in the trap of preferring running as my regular exercise. In doing so, however, it limits the diversity of muscle use. Even though I can have a very efficient cardiac output, I have more difficulty playing other sports requiring use of other muscles. I need to train all my muscles to have the healthiest body. If I would play a round of tennis for an hour after not playing it for a year, I would notice soreness because my muscles are not accustomed to handling that intensity of use. Similarly, the ingestion of a diversity of fiber would initially lead to some initial intestinal discomfort and gas. Overtime gradually ramping up with dietary training it is well tolerated as the abundance of a healthy microbiome in our intestines is created.

SCFAs affect local health right at the intestinal level leading to stronger junctions in the intestinal cells and less inflammation. Butyrate has been especially useful in restoring the tight junctions in the colon cells. This helps prevent "leaky gut." The SCFAs are the primary source of energy for our colon cells, making up 70% of their energy. In fact, 10% of our energy is met with fiber derived SCFAs when we eat a WFPBD.

A leaky gut means the intestinal cell junctions are more permeable, with holes allowing bacteria and endotoxins to pass through the intestinal wall to activate the immune system in an inappropriate way leading to local and systemic inflammation. Butyrate increases the production of proteins that maintain healthy connections between the cells. Think about it like the children's game Red Rover where children link arms so that the person running can't break through easily. The stronger the colon links, the harder it is for bad actors to get through.

Also, butyrate has been shown to increase colonic motility and decrease gut hypersensitivity. As we have learned about earlier, those with FM-like pain disorders like IBS are about twice as sensitive as those without IBS. They report pain triggered at half the intestinal air pressure as those without IBS.

SCFAs
- The dominant energy source for healthy bacteria
- Repair leaky gut
- Reduce bacterial endotoxin release
- Promotes motility
- Decrease visceral (gut) sensitivity

When the barrier is broken down in diseases like Crohn's, E. coli invades the lining, and the immune system attacks the bacteria. The attack causes collateral damage to the intestines.

Those with Crohn's disease also are more likely to have IBS. What happens when a diet high in fiber is used to treat Crohn's disease? Those on the semi-vegetarian diet maintained a 92 percent remission rate compared to 33% among omnivores. A WFPB also was shown to improve rheumatoid arthritis symptoms in 41% of patients compared to 4% on a general diet. It is incredible to think about how interconnected and intricate our bodies are, and the impact food has on our well-being.

The SCFAs get absorbed and act regionally within the intestinal system affecting satiety in the stomach. The SCFAs stimulate G coupled receptors that were considered orphan receptors because they, for a long time, had unknown "keys" to unlock them.

Painful stimuli such as distention of the bowels is sensed by pain receptors, expressed at the intestinal nerve terminations, project signals onto the spinal cord. These take the signals through the spinal cord to the brain and brainstem. Here, the signal reaches several brain areas. These include the thalamus, hypothalamus, limbic system, and cortex. The signals from the intestines are interpreted and a signal is sent back to the intestines. These signals help manage the rate food is pushed through the intestines.

From the gut, the microbiota can communicate with the central nervous system (CNS), forming complex crosstalk between the gut, its microbiome, and the brain known as the microbiota-gut-brain (MGB) axis.

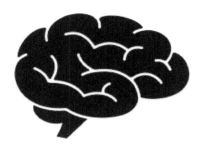

Gut brain axis:
Back and forth
communication

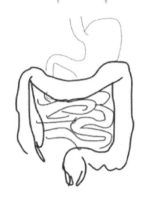

This bidirectional communication between the gut microbiota and the brain is believed to help regulate gastrointestinal homeostasis, also known as a balance. This affects mood, thinking, and pain perception.

SCFAs also affect blood sugar regulation. A high-fiber diet promotes healthy bacteria that regulate blood glucose control in complex ways.

Second Meal Effect

The second meal effect occurs when glucose control changes if the meal eaten 5 hours earlier was high fiber such as lentils through the release of SCFAs. This effect happens because the stomach emptying time is slowed down, decreasing how fast the food enters the small intestines where most glucose is absorbed. Because many who have fibromyalgia struggle with obesity and impulsive eating, activating your natural satiety pathways through consuming a diet high in fiber makes it much easier to bypass your susceptibility to calorie-dense, low, or fiber-free comfort food.

Why rely on will power alone to adhere to a typical portion control standard American diet that is doomed to fail? The average American diet is low in fiber compared to a whole-foods plant-based fiber naturally high in fiber. Over time, with adoption of a whole-foods plant-based diet, the cravings go away as you are not starving yourself of calories. And you were fending off real hunger only to cycle back to gaining weight when you don't have the natural appetite suppression feedback through SCFAs produced from the fiber-rich diet you now consume.

You will also feel more energy after dinner. How often have you had good exercise intentions go to waste after dinner because you fall into a "food coma?" Instead, now free of the diet dragging you down, you are activated and complete your exercise goals with much less effort. Furthermore, the microbiota is believed to influence function and metabolism of gut hormone cells, inducing the expression of several peptides, such as glucagon-like peptides (GLP) and peptide YY (PYY), which are known to control energy balance, glucose metabolism, gut barrier function, and metabolic inflammation.

Brain Fog Improvement with Diet

SCFAs, such as butyrate, improve the health of the barrier between our blood and brain. This leads to improved learning and memory. Lab studies have demonstrated the protective effect of SCFAs on amyloid plaque formation, which is characteristic of Alzheimer's. Children on high-fiber diets improve multitasking, working memory, and focus compared to those on a low fiber diet. There also may be a connection with Parkinson's disease.

The microbiota is also capable of regulating the production and release of several neurotransmitters in the Intestinal tract. Serotonin release though bacteria in the intestines has been to be involved in colonic function and GI disorders. For instance, lower levels of serotonin and building blocks along with serotonin reuptake transporter (SERT) expression levels have been reported in some studies involving IBS patients.

Eating a Western diet low in fiber takes about two to four days for the food you eat to exit your body compared to 18-24 hours on a whole-foods plant-based diet. Other neurotransmitters γ-aminobutyric acid (GABA), dopamine (DA) and acetylcholine (ACh) are synthesized inside the intestinal cavity by the microbiota which are believed to communicate with the brain through the gut brain axis.

If you're genetically prone to lower levels of these neurotransmitters, you have a greater need to feed the bacteria fiber that will lead to increased levels. This is similar to how you need more exercise than the person unaffected by FM-like pain to feel the best.

The role bacteria play in signaling within the nervous system of the gut has been shown in several experiments. You can experimentally raise mice without bacteria in their intestines resulting in higher weight. These mice have abnormal functioning of their nervous system. By giving the microbiota from healthy mice to the germ-free mice, restoration of normal excitability of gut sensory neurons occurs. A fecal transplant from IBS patients reproduced certain features of IBS in germ-free mice, including hypersensitivity to colorectal distention.

Intestinal dysbiosis (unhealthy bacterial makeup) has also been reported in individuals suffering from visceral pain, including IBS patients, making the microbiota itself a novel target for treatment. A reduction in the levels of Bifidobacterium, Lactobacillus, and alterations in the Firmicutes: Bacteroidetes ratio, which represents the most abundant bacteria family found within the human gut microbiome, have been identified in IBS patients.

Which diet promotes a healthy Firmicute: Bacteroides ratio?

A diet high in fiber and low in processed carbs that have been stripped of fiber does. A diet that is high in oils and carbs that also are devoid of fiber promotes an unhealthy ratio. This healthy ratio is precisely what a whole-foods plant-based diet with minimally added fat contains. These mechanisms explain the basis for the dramatic reductions in pain the low-fat whole-foods plant-based diet achieved.

What is the most prominent predictor of a healthy gut microbiome?

The diversity of plants in one's diet.

Having 30 or more different plants was more important, whether or not you said you were vegan. You could be a junk food vegan who just doesn't eat meat or dairy but has a tiny amount of whole, unprocessed, plant foods. A style of Paleo diet that has broad diversity and a large number of whole plants would be healthier than the junk food vegan diet.

A whole-foods plant-based diet also leads to steady weight loss.

Weight loss can have a big reduction on pain and fibromyalgia symptoms.

A study of intensive weight loss with diet and exercise on the effects of knee pain showed impressive reductions in pain. Whether inflammation constitutes a separate osteoarthritis (OA) disease pathway or instead is the downstream result of chronic excessive biomechanical stress is debated. Systemic inflammation markers, including Interleukin-6 (IL-6), distinguished patients with knee or hip OA from controls, and higher systemic levels of IL-6 have been associated with increased odds of developing knee OA.

Diffusion of such inflammatory proteins from the joint fluid into the cartilage could contribute to cartilage matrix loss by stimulating the breakdown of cartilage and inhibiting growth. In addition to these direct effects on the joint, inflammatory mediators can affect muscle function and lower the pain threshold. IL-6 concentrations less than 2.5 pg/mL have been shown to reduce the risk of mobility disability and improve markers of metabolic syndrome. Pain was reduced the greatest in the diet and exercise group.

Himann et al. found that walking speed decreased by 1% to 2% per decade of adult life until age 62 when the decline was 12% to 16% per decade. The demonstrated reversal of this trend by increasing their walking speed and 6-minute walk distance, diet changes, and increased exercise participation was significantly more than the exercise alone and diet alone groups. These improvements, in part, may have been due to the significant reduction in knee pain. Independent of group assignment, participants who lost 10% or more of body weight improved function and reduced knee compressive force, systemic IL-6 concentrations, and pain more than those who lost 5% to 9.9% or less than 5% of their baseline weight.

It is not uncommon for me to see patients who have well over the 10% excess of their ideal body weight, often over 100 lbs. If you are 200 lbs. and your ideal bodyweight is 160 lbs., then losing half of the weight to 21 or more pounds puts you in the 10%+ category. There are exciting opportunities for improvement in pain if that describes you. If you are in this category or know someone who is, seriously consider encouraging them to move in the direction of a low-fat whole-foods plant-based diet.

Inflammation levels measured by high sensitivity C-reactive protein also decrease with a low-fat whole-foods plant-based diet. Studies are suggesting decreased autoimmune activity with diseases like rheumatoid arthritis, lupus, and multiple sclerosis. As mentioned earlier, diet also affects Crohn's disease with higher levels of animal protein increasing the risk of development. A semi-vegetarian diet was very effective in preventing relapse of Crohn's disease. There also is a decreased pain signaling from intestinal nerve sensors contributing to less overall pain.

Less inflammation also leads to increased mobility. The increasing levels of exercise lead to regression of pain.

Besides improvement in knee pain alone with weight loss through diet and exercise, other areas of the body pain lessen through diet and exercise. Diffuse pain is found with fibromyalgia. This improvement was demonstrated by a study by Dr. Daniel Clauw using an 800-calorie diet with meal replacements and moderate exercise. This study's chief finding is that following weight loss induced by a low-calorie diet, the spatial distribution of pain and somatic symptoms improved, two hallmarks of complex chronic pain conditions. The total number of areas were reduced, and general symptoms of bodily pain were reduced. These results appear to be the serendipitous result of weight loss, as the participants did not seek treatment for general body pain.

After the intervention, fewer individuals had pain in weight-bearing areas like the lower back and lower leg, as noted in many previous studies. There was also some improvement in non-weight-bearing regions like the jaw, chest, and abdomen. These patterns were not consistent with a simple global reduction in pain but seemed to vary by the site as there was some pattern of worsening in the upper back, neck, and shoulders. In addition to the composite measure of symptom severity (i.e., fatigue, sleep difficulties), depression scores improved substantially.

Those who lost more than 10% of their initial body weight showed a more remarkable improvement in depression, pain, and total modified ACR scores (a measurement of arthritis symptoms). Over four-tenths of those who lost greater than 10% of their body weight showed at least a 30% reduction in ACR (American College of Rheumatology) pain scores, a metric that corresponds well with other pain measures and with patients' ratings of "much improved."

Unfortunately, long term adherence to meal replacement diets and major calorie restricted diets used in this study are in real life and for long term a challenge and really not sustainable for most.

However, the implementation of a whole-food plant-based diet shows long term weight loss success and palatability. Implementation of a WFPBD can lead to weight loss. Weight loss has been shown to decrease pain markedly but has been for many challenging to maintain. Studies show that long-term adherence to a low-fat whole-foods plant-based diet is very effective. Compliance occurs because there is true satiety that arises because of the feedback mechanisms through the signaling of short-chain fatty acid production to the stomach and brain. Also, unprocessed fiber-containing foods, AKA whole plants, stretch the stomach receptors giving the fullness feeling with fewer calories. Food with fiber gets to the end of the small intestine, and the "ileal brake" is activated, signaling to the brain satiety. I will share more of the details later.

Neal Barnard's diabetes study showed a higher level of satisfaction with a low-fat whole-foods plant-based diet compared to the carb counting traditional diabetes diet, as well as better diabetes, blood pressure, and cholesterol control.

Adherence can additionally be a challenge as many with chronic pain are accustomed to a very calorie-dense diet of salt, sugar and fat, and is very low in fiber. Problems include the addictive quality of foods high in fat, salt, and processed carbs; cultural influences of marketing, our family upbringings, and choices in restaurants; and knowing what to substitute in place of these unhealthy foods. These have an addictive-like effect giving short term pleasure but lead to weight gain and worsening pain and inflammation.

Foods that turn to sugar quickly affect the same part of the brain as cocaine. Cheese and chocolate affect the same part of the brain as morphine. It is not uncommon for those who change to a low-fat whole-foods plant-based diet to have some withdrawal symptoms. This is typically replaced relatively quickly by feeling better.

If you have the added burden of untreated ADHD, which occurs in about half or more of people with fibromyalgia, you then carry even a greater barrier to sticking with a whole-food plant-based diet. ADHD makes it harder to lose weight and adhere to a WFPD diet. You are more susceptible to impulsive eating and food choices when shopping. You are less likely to plan your meals. Untreated ADHD also increases the risk of developing diabetes by 50%.

Fortunately, ADHD can be treated with medicine, learning coping strategies, and partnering with someone like a dietitian trained in this area. Teaming up with a family member is also an opportunity to reinforce your new choices, but they could also undermine your efforts. One of the purposes of this book has been to educate you and your family members. I am all too aware of how prickly your family can be around individual food choices and not wanting to be told what to do or change. If you have had fibromyalgia for years, doing the same thing, including your eating habits, hasn't helped. Why not try something that is helpful and has minimal, if any, adverse secondary effects when initiated gradually?

Cardiovascular Disease Reversal with a Plant-based Diet

A healthy heart and blood vessels increase greater exercise capacity and lead to improved symptoms of fibromyalgia.

If you have shortness of breath with walking due to blockages in the arteries or diminished pumping capacity of your heart, you will have significant restrictions on your exercise capacities. Exercise is so beneficial by activating the pain inhibition areas of the nervous system. However, if we could improve the blood flow of your arteries to your heart and skeletal muscles, you could exercise more. When your heart pumps more effectively, you increase your exercise capacity as well. A whole-food plant-based diet (WFPBD) is the only diet that has been shown to reverse blood flow in the arteries of the heart.

Blood flow with a WFPBD has also been demonstrated to improve in two studies. Drs. Caldwell Esselstyn and Dean Ornish have demonstrated reversal of heart disease on a low-fat whole-foods plant-based diet. The blockages in arteries, known as arteriosclerosis, showed reversal as well as improved blood flow on cardiac stress tests. The artery walls become more compliant leading to blood pressure reductions to healthy levels. Blood flow to the arteries of the legs also has shown reversal. These can lead to fewer difficulties with exercise. Exercise is vital for reducing the symptoms of fibromyalgia.

Dr. Peter Linn, a vascular surgeon, demonstrated a whole-foods plant-based diet that improved vascular endothelial function in patients with peripheral artery disease, (blockages in the leg arteries) following four months of dietary intervention. The endothelial cells are the cells lining the arteries and are very important in controlling the healthy function of the arteries. This dietary intervention also resulted in decreased serum cholesterol and inflammatory biomarkers, which may further enhance vascular endothelial function.

Unfortunately, if you are like most people, you are not eating a WFPBD. **Studies show that those with chronic pain, compared to those without, eat an unhealthy diet. They are twice as likely to eat fruits or vegetables less than once a week and are more likely to eat fatty food, chips, or French fries.**

Why is that? There are several reasons to explore.

The Pleasure Trap

"Dr. Lenz, I know it makes sense to eat a Whole-Foods plant-based diet, I don't doubt it at all, but I just don't find the food very delicious. It doesn't taste good. I don't like vegetables, beans, or fruit very much."

I hear this often and it is similar to working with other addictions like smoking. You can, however, learn to not just like the food, but actually love it and strongly prefer eating a whole-plant food-based diet. What would you say to someone who struggled with quitting smoking and couldn't understand why they couldn't quit? The answer is the powerfully addictive effect of nicotine. It hits the part of the brain that gives the feeling that "everything is ok." Withdrawal gives the complete opposite feeling, everything doesn't "feel ok."

But why do you love the diet of cheese, meats, and processed carbs with added oils, salts, and fats? Our bodies are designed to function optimally on a whole-foods plant-based diet but our hunger signals and satiety can be hijacked. When foods that turn to sugar quickly, a large burst of dopamine is released in the pleasure center of the brain. This is the same center that is activated by cocaine.

Studies have shown that at the neurobiological level, the effects of sugar on the reward centers of the brain may be more robust than those of cocaine. In addition, studies have found that heavy users of sugar develop tolerance (needing more and more to feel the same effect), which is a symptom of substance dependence. Foods higher in fat and dairy, especially cheese, hit the opioid receptors of the brain. Chocolate, especially with added sugar and fat, also hits the opioid reward center.

Supranormal Stimulus

A supranormal stimulus is a term used to describe any stimulus that elicits a response stronger than the stimulus for which it is designed, even if it is artificial. Sources of "super" stimulation like junk food give a more intense response to the reward center of the brain. Examples of food with supranormal stimuli include French fries, cheese, hamburger, chips, chocolate, pizza, donuts, and ice cream.

Step 1- You eat medium to low calorie density food and have a moderate amount of pleasure. Think of the medium pleasure is the area of a low to moderate calorie density of whole grains, fruits, vegetables, legumes.

Step 2- Doing the wrong thing feels right. You eat the calorie dense foods, and it is very pleasurable. It is very rewarding. It tastes better to you. This also applies to other addictions like cocaine addiction.

Step 3- The pleasure subsides after eating the calorie dense foods.

Step 4- You are back to your baseline. Hunger begins to grow.

Step 5- You try a whole-foods plant-based recipe that is naturally less calorie dense. It actually doesn't taste good to you.

Step 6- After eating a plant-based diet drops the pleasure set point.

Step 7 - Eating a whole-foods plant-based diet starts to taste good.

Food companies know the pleasure trap well, and they manipulate the levels of salt, sugar, and fat to get people hooked on them. Food companies try to optimize this by reaching the bliss point. The bliss point is the combination of an ingredient such as salt, sugar, or fat which optimizes the taste. Michael Moss details these in his book, *Salt Sugar Fat: How the Food Giants Hooked Us*. When they act in concert, they are more rewarding than any one alone.

Once hooked, more and more are needed to get the same level of satisfaction. Without eating the fiber to naturally suppress appetite we will learn more about, one is accustomed to having unnaturally high dopamine stimulation. The body protects itself by lowering the number of dopamine receptors. At this level, foods that give pleasure, like an apple without caramel, actually taste bad.

A simple analogy is eating apples. In the past I would eat apples in the Fall. The first week I might get a dozen apples and eat them over a week. The next week when I go shopping, I see the caramel apples and tubs of caramel dip strategically placed next to the regular apples. I think, "hey, you deserve a treat," and get the caramel dip with the apples and the caramel and M and M covered apples to treat myself. After eating those for a week, I go back to eating regular apples. They don't taste as good now, with the sweetness like celery.

Restrict your diet to vegetables and water for several days or 2 weeks and see what happens. When fruit is introduced you will report it as the sweetest apple you have ever had in your life. Temporary restrictions like these are known as fasting mimicking diets but have to be done carefully and activity should be limited during those times.

This applies to so many other foods and recipes you commonly eat including foods such as a vegetable salad with chicken, croutons, cheese, eggs, and a fatty salad dressing like ranch. Eating the same salad but substituting beans, quinoa, avocados, and vinegar or lime juice will be rated a lot less appealing initially. Overtime with adoption of a no added fat whole-foods plant-based diet, however, the food will become much tastier and the fatty salad will actually be too intense and not enjoyable. If you drink soda regularly, water doesn't taste very good, but if you drink water as your only beverage and then drink a soda it will feel too sweet and unappealing. Do you enjoy coffee or beer? If you do it is likely that when you first tasted it, you thought it was very bitter but acquired a taste for it over time.

I was interviewed by a local news station when Michelle Obama came to nearby Watertown, Wisconsin during her campaign to encourage drinking water. Just like First Lady Barbara Bush encouraged reading books, who can argue with drinking water? Drinking water does definitely have health benefits, one of which is that you are not drinking soda or other sugary fiber free beverages.

What she couldn't say publicly for political reasons, is don't drink soda. This is similar to diet advice. Someone eating the typical American diet is somewhat ok with being told to eat more fruits and vegetables, but tell them to stop eating meats, dairy, processed carbs and added fats and then the heels get dug in and defenses go up. It is also very difficult to say as a public official to speak against the ill effects of non-whole plant foods due to the huge agribusiness economy. It is a very sensitive issue. Tell a patient that the chronic use of opioids for their FM is making their symptoms worse and you will get a similar reaction. More on that in a subsequent chapter.

A few ideas to accelerate the transition from calorie dense food:
- Fasting or a fasting mimicking diet.

- Unlimited amounts of legumes and vegetables only for 5 days. Drink lots of water
- "Go to jail" Do a self-imposed 48-hour water fast. Longer durations would have to be medically supervised or at least done very carefully.

In addition, to the food being addicting, culture has a big influence. We are heavily marketed the bad food which is consumed by the majority of people that we are around. Your family and friends all eat this way which can be very challenging. This is similar to smoking. In the 1960s there were hundreds of studies showing the damage and addictive qualities of cigarettes, but it continued to be common practice. I still have patients who struggle with smoking cessation, but it isn't due to a lack of awareness of the poor health and addictive qualities of smoking. Some get mad at themselves and say, "Why can't I quit, it's just a cigarette?"

Slowly, this awareness of the addictive qualities of food is occurring. Studies and clinical experience have shown that quitting smoking cold turkey is more effective than slowly weaning off. If you still have some cigarettes and have a stressful day, you can always get some momentary relief. Asking someone who smokes, "why do you continue smoking? Don't you know it's so unhealthy?" "I know it is unhealthy, but I have 20 friends in my pocket, and they are always there for me." This principal also applies to food. "When I am stressed, the cheeseburger, French fries, ice cream, bacon, candy, etc., are always there for me. That's how I cope with stress."

In the next section we will talk about the implementation of eating a whole-foods plant-based diet. You will become more equipped to make the lifestyle changes.

I often hear, and you may be thinking, "Doc, there's a big difference between eating and smoking. I don't have to smoke, but I do have to eat." My response is that you do have to eat, but you don't have to eat the calorie dense addictive foods. You can choose to eat healthy foods. Trust me when I tell you that over time your taste buds will change to enjoying plant-based foods. You will be surprised how good the food will taste over time when you avoid the unhealthy food.

Admittedly, it is in many ways easier to quit smoking due to several reasons. There is social discouragement to smoke and eat a whole-foods plant-based diet. However, there is encouragement to quit smoking and eat a calorie dense diet. This is slowly changing but may take decades to change, similar to how our social perception of smoking took decades to change.

Are You "Chemically Wired" to Gain Weight?

If, however, you have untreated ADHD, you are more susceptible to poor diet choices. ADHD treatment generally causes some weight loss, but more importantly, it levels the playing field. It makes you just as susceptible to the addictive foods as everyone else, not more susceptible like one with untreated ADHD is. Those with ADHD often fall into the trap of *"procrastineating"* which is eating calorie dense pleasure foods to de-stress in place of doing work requiring a lot of focus, planning, organization, and patience.

Impulsive or disordered eating and unplanned meals are partially to blame for ADHD's strong correlation with obesity. And then there's your dopamine-seeking brain, which loves refined carbs, salt, and fat. What you may not know is that excessive body weight is disproportionately prevalent among people who have ADHD. And, given their impulsivity and their often-erratic eating habits, people with ADHD have an unusually difficult time losing excess weight once they've gained it. I have observed this in numerous obese patients with untreated ADHD. A 2005 study revealed that the rate of ADHD was five to 10 times greater among these overweight individuals than in the general population (30 percent versus 3 to 6 percent).

We will now talk about how a whole-foods plant-based diet works, but keep in mind that after you learn how it works and how to implement it, it doesn't mean you will do it. I will share further insight on what may be sabotaging you to eating healthy.

How eating a whole-foods plant-based diet works:

Step 1- Stomach fullness

Is a calorie just a calorie? Are 100 calories of carrots the same as 100 calories of cola? You could consume cola calories very quickly compared to the much longer amount of time it would take to eat the same number of Calories in carrots. Traditional diets involve cutting calories. A 2-week study looked at comparing the effect of identical amounts of calories between two diets over 2 weeks in a hospital-controlled study. One was ultra-processed foods like a white bread sandwich with meat, baked potato chips, sugar free soda and yogurt. The other was a whole-foods plant-based diet. The ultra-processed group gained 2 lbs. on average over the 2 weeks and the whole-foods plant-based diet group lost 2 lbs. A simple remedy to the standard American diet of ultra-processed plants and animal protein is to take away the added fat and add the vegetables, greens, whole intact grains, and legumes.

Stomach distension makes you feel full when you have food that contains water and fiber naturally. Increased stretching of the stomach with lower calories leads to satiety. You feel fuller on fewer calories. Many have claimed that weight loss with a plant-based diet occurs because one just eats fewer calories. This is true because ad lib calorie intake of a low-fat whole plant food is less than the standard western diet. However, in one study, subjects were force fed about an extra 500 Calories to make up for the difference and they still lost weight. This is likely due to the thermogenic effect of food where the metabolism of a WFPBD burns more calories.

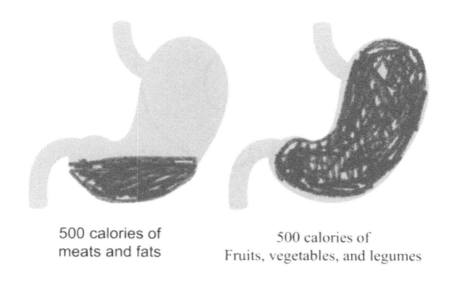

500 calories of
meats and fats

500 calories of
Fruits, vegetables, and legumes

It is better to eat food that has water in it. Whole cooked oat groats contain a much higher amount of water compared to dry cereal and fills you up more than twice as much. The more water in the food the greater satiety you will have.

Step 2- Ileal Brake
When food contains fiber the digestion of carbohydrates continues to the end of the small intestine known as the ileum.

This sends a signal to the brain stimulating a decrease in appetite. If a whole plant food is ultra-processed, meaning nearly all the fiber is removed, the carbohydrates get absorbed in the first part of the intestines known as the duodenum and never get to the ileum to trigger the satiety signal.

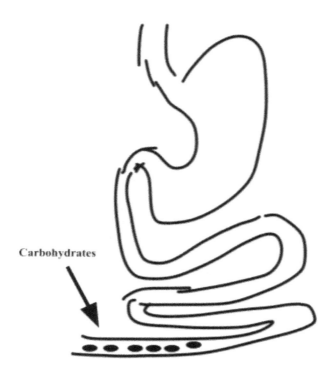

Carbohydrates

Part 3 Postbiotics
Fiber leads to the production of chemical compounds known as postbiotics that have profound effects on health. When whole plant food is eaten the stomach and small intestine absorb vital nutrients. What is left is fiber, which used to be considered as unessential. This mistaken understanding was

why companies thought they could remove it from flour and not have any harms. Subsequent discoveries have uncovered an incredibly intricate design with a satiety feedback to the brain. Fiber is left over from food after it leaves the small intestines and enters the colon. Fiber is processed by the healthy bacteria in the intestines that not only keep the bacteria healthy but us as well, known as symbiotic relationship. The huge variety of bacteria act as chemical processing and manufacturing centers by producing short chain fatty acids (SCFAs) and building blocks for neurotransmitters that are used to signal between neurons.

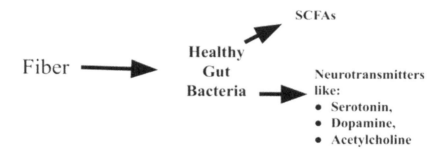

Short chain fatty acids (SCFAs) have profound effects including communicating fullness to the brain and telling the stomach to empty slower. They also keep the colon cells healthy by feeding them and making sure the immune system works properly.

Building blocks for neurotransmitters are produced for serotonin, dopamine, and acetylcholine among others that contribute to the "feeling good" that one experiences with eating a whole-foods plant-based diet.

Butyrates, an SCFA, has been found to be an effective IBS therapy. To date, a few trials have been performed to evaluate the effectiveness of sodium butyrate on clinical symptoms and quality of life in patients with IBS. Banasiewicz *et al.* performed a double-blind, randomized, placebo-controlled study in which 66 adult patients with IBS received microencapsulated butyric acid at a dose of 300 mg per day or placebo as an adjunct to standard therapy. At four weeks, the frequency of abdominal pain during defecation in the butyric acid group was noticeably less.

At 12 weeks, decreases in the frequency of spontaneous abdominal pain, postprandial abdominal pain, abdominal pain during defecation and urge after defecation were observed. Butyrates are not available by prescription but are available when you feed fiber to the butyrate producing bacteria in your colon. In other words, eat the food that contains fiber.

Willpower

You may have thought that you don't have the willpower to eat a plant-based diet. I have heard many people ask if I have strong cravings to eat the calorie dense foods. I actually don't, and here is a study to support how the effects of eating a whole plant-based diet makes it easy to do. Researchers investigated the effect of increased colonic propionate (a SCFA) production on brain anticipatory reward responses during food picture evaluation.

Researchers hypothesized that elevated colonic propionate would reduce both reward responses and ad libitum energy intake via stimulation of anorexigenic (appetite suppressing) gut hormone secretion. 20 healthy nonobese men completed a functional magnetic resonance imaging (fMRI) food picture evaluation task after consumption of control inulin or inulin-propionate ester, a unique dietary compound that selectively augments colonic propionate production.

The blood oxygen level dependent (BOLD) signal was measured in brain regions known to be involved in reward processing, including the caudate, nucleus accumbens, amygdala, anterior insula, and orbitofrontal cortex. Increasing colonic propionate production reduced BOLD signal during food picture evaluation in the caudate and nucleus accumbens. In the caudate, the reduction in BOLD signal was driven specifically by a lowering of the response to high-energy food. These effects on the brain were partnered with a decrease in subjective appeal of high-energy food pictures and reduced energy intake during an ad libitum meal.

12-Week Plant-Based Dietary Intervention

In 2017 a group in New Zealand did a study looking at empowerment by informing those in the intervention group about a whole-foods plant-based diet. There were no restrictions of healthy foods and over 12 weeks of the study they lost 19 lbs. on average. After that no more instruction was given. It takes about 12 weeks for an intentional behavior to become cemented into a habit. Six months later they lost another 27 pounds. They had felt so much better that they continued with the diet changes and the weight came off. A year later they maintained the weight loss.

The most common advice given to those on a traditional western diet is to just reduce the portions of the same foods. 95% or more people who eat the same kinds of the standard American diet, but smaller portions will gain all the weight they lost in the first 6 months within 12 months. A portion control diet with the traditional low fiber, calorie dense Western diet is set up to fail. On a whole-foods plant-based diet there is no restriction in the quantity of foods one is allowed to eat. People consume less calories on a WFPB diet, feel full, have more energy, lose weight, and have less pain.

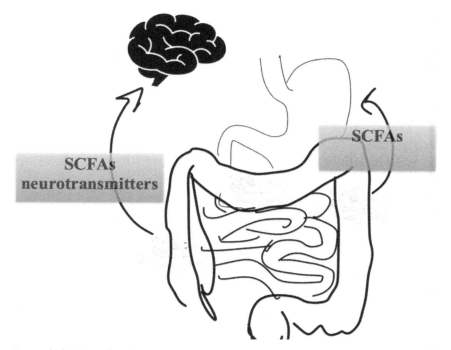

Bacteria in the colon digest fiber to produce essential compounds that feedback to the brain and stomach signaling satiety.

Why doesn't portion control work?

"All you need to do is cut your portions." You have likely tried that, but it doesn't work. It doesn't work because your body doesn't get the satiety signal. You can eat less but not be satisfied. In the short term you can "will power" it out, but in the long term it doesn't work. It is easy to lose weight this way for 6 months but 1 year, 3 years, and 10 years later that weight and more is gained back.

In addition, the calorie dense, fiber depleted food gives an immediate reward signal to the brain and an immediate rush of pleasure through the release of dopamine. This leads to a diminished enjoyment of the whole plant foods and an addiction like bond with the calorie dense foods as was discussed earlier in the discussion on the "pleasure trap."

How should you consider undertaking diet changes?

Plan, Practice, and Persist
1. **Create a simple plan.**
2. **Practice**
3. **Persist by adding variety.**

Create a simple meal plan revolving around easy recipes and foods you already enjoy or at least somewhat enjoy. You likely will have to do some adjustments.

Meals like oatmeal or baked potato or stir fry with brown rice and vegetables. Many of you have eaten plant-based recipes much of your life but did not consider them plant based. Spaghetti with marinara sauce, lentils, peppers, onions, mushrooms, and zucchini for example. A whole wheat burrito with beans, steamed sweet potatoes, onions, tomatoes, lettuce, onions and guacamole.

Recipes

I want to give you some relatively easy meal ideas that you can use and then expand from there.

Start your day with a healthy breakfast.

For many these are easy because you likely only are preparing food for yourself and don't have the social pressures of eating with others who may not be on the WFPBD train just yet. A great breakfast and one I eat most of the time is some whole cooked grain with fruit. Most often this is either oat groats I make in the instant pot or traditional oatmeal. I vary on what fruits I add.

Monday- oat groats with bananas and walnuts. I take 1 cup of oats and 2.5 cups of water and set it to grains and cook for 23 minutes. I might make extra and store them for a couple days so I can just save time and reheat it in the microwave the next day.

Tuesday- traditional oatmeal with strawberries

Wednesday- Oatmeal with mangos and a tablespoon of cocoa powder

Thursday- Oats with frozen mixed berries that I thawed out.

Friday- Oats with frozen cherries and cocoa powder

On the weekend I might have more time.

Saturday- Whole wheat waffles made with applesauce and flaxseed in place of oil and eggs. I will add fruit on top in place of butter and syrup.

Sunday- a breakfast burrito made with steamed veggies, salsa and tofu/ or other beans.

If you are thinking that this is boring or don't like oatmeal, let's think about that. How often do you eat sandwiches with bread and meat with slight variations every day for lunch? Which is more boring? If you don't think you like oatmeal due to the texture, I didn't either until a few years ago. It was a hang-up since childhood when oatmeal reminded me of baby food that my baby sister was eating. And compared to eating processed sugar cereal, oats tasted like cardboard. What's great about breakfast like these options is that they are easy and quick. They also keep you full for many hours. It is not uncommon that a breakfast for me of a cup of dry oatmeal with a couple bananas and walnuts would keep me full for several hours from 7 Am to 2 PM if needed during a busy clinic day.

If you still have a hang up with oatmeal, consider maybe a half cup of oatmeal with 2 cups of fruit and then gradually increase the portion of oats over time.

Lunch

A simple tip is to eat leftovers from your supper the night before. Also, it is good to batch cook on days off so you can save time during the week. Batch cooking is simply the act of preparing and/or cooking larger portions of different foods, meant to be mixed and matched to create versatile meals throughout the week. It's typically done on a Sunday, to prepare for the week ahead.

Lunch also tends to be easier because most people eat by themselves, so they are less likely to be tempted by calorie dense foods others are eating. Of course, if you are taking clients out for lunch, you have to be more determined and confident with your choices.

Batch cook or prep the following items to have ready during the week.

- Diced or sliced onions
- Cut or diced peppers of different varieties
- Cube sweet potatoes, squash, and eggplant that have been roasted with spiced vinegar glaze
- Broccoli and cauliflower
- Diced tomatoes
- Diced cucumbers

Lunch Ideas

- Whole wheat pasta with fat free and no added sugar marinara sauce with lentils. Add some other vegetables if you like.
- Tortilla with fat free refried black beans or pinto beans with salsa. Add some onions, sweet potatoes and peppers as you like
- Quinoa bowl with black beans, roasted eggplant and squash, shredded red cabbage and carrots, roasted sweet potatoes, chopped leek and spinach. Cover with a peanut dressing made with vinegar, ginger, cayenne pepper, soy sauce and a small amount of peanut butter
- Leftover whole wheat veggies pizza

What's for dessert?
Fruits are for dessert with unlimited variety and quantity.

What should I snack on?
For most people, snacks are not necessary unless you are exercising at a very high level or going through puberty. Snacks are more likely consumed for most people because you are stressed to some degree and are eating the calorie dense nutritionally depleted foods compared to a WFPBD. This includes processed carbs full of salt, foods that turn to sugar quickly, and fat.

Also, may be higher in fat like cheese and meats. Also, if you are truly hungry it may be that a banana was just not enough to cut it. You need to eat oatmeal with it along with 2 bananas and some walnuts for example. The volume of your food will be higher. You are likely conditioned to think the higher volume of food is too much and you need to watch your portions. What's great about eating this way is that you don't have to count your portions or calories.

Plant-Based Pantry List

- **Beans**- black, cannellini, chickpeas (garbanzo), kidney, lima, pinto. Canned beans are more convenient but if you have time or a pressure cooker dry beans are great.
- **Lentils black, red, green or brown**
- **Beets no added sugar**
- **Brown rice or wild rice or black rice**
- **Applesauce (used in baking)**
- **Dried fruit: dates, raisins, apricots or other, unsweetened**
- **Nuts unsalted and raw (almonds, cashews, pecans, walnuts)**
- **Nut butter almond butter or natural peanut butter, no added sugar or oil**
- **Oats** (steel cut or rolled, whole)
- **Quinoa**
- **Canned tomatoes** diced
- **Tubers and starchy vegetables** (potatoes, sweet potatoes, winter squash)
- **Vegetable broth** low sodium if desired
- **Vinegars:** apple cider vinegar. Aged vinegars, specialty vinegars and a local vinegar store, balsamic, and natural rice

Freezer list:

- **Frozen fruit**
- **Frozen vegetables (corn and peas and edamame in particular)**

Refrigerator list:

- **Non-dairy milk almond, cashew, coconut, or soy milk**

- Tofu/tempeh
- Seeds flax, chia, hemp, sunflower seeds
- Tahini
- Pure Maple syrup
- Dijon mustard
- Nutritional yeast
- Soy Sauce (or Bragg Liquid Aminos, low sodium if you prefer)

Whole wheat/grain breads:

Crackers (low fat) and pasta

Fruit and Veggie ideas:

Bananas, Berries, Grapes, particularly red or black, Lemons/limes, Pineapple Carrots, Broccoli, Cauliflower

Green Leafy Vegetables:
Romaine, Mesclun, Red Leaf Lettuce, Baby Greens, Spinach, and Broccoli Sprouts, dark green leafy vegetables Asparagus, Arugula, Beets, Beet Greens, Broccoli Rabe, Bok Choy, Brussels Sprouts, Cabbage, Chicory, Cilantro, Collard Greens, Endive, Kale (Curly or Lacinato), Microgreens, Mustard Greens, Parsley, Spinach, Sweet Potato Leaves, Swiss Chard, Turnip Greens and Watercress.

Unfiltered Extra Virgin Olive Oil to use sparingly or skip.

Organic Canola Oil to use sparingly or skip

Meal Planning

Is it expensive and hard to eat a plant-based diet? Your choices are varied from cheap to expensive standard

American food. The same is for a whole-foods plant-based diet. The food can be simple or gourmet.

Keep in mind that just trying a few meals the first week is a good start for most. Maybe oatmeal with fruit for breakfast, a burrito with vegetables, beans and guacamole; or pasta with roasted vegetables and lentils with a delicious marinara sauce. There are many resources available. Consider working with a dietitian. Some are available online through programs to guide you on this transformation.

Go to the www.plantrician.org website to find one in your area. Remember the benefits you will get as you adopt these changes. Envision feeling better with less constipation, bloating, headaches, and body pains. Imagine climbing stairs easier and going on long walks.

Persistence

As you start to feel better, you will likely want to add more healthy foods to your diet. If you also have coexisting medical problems like diabetes and high blood pressure, you will see significant changes, often happening within days. The effects on your blood pressure and diabetes can be so powerful that within days your blood sugars and blood pressure can drop. Make sure you monitor your levels frequently if you are on medications as hypoglycemia and low blood pressure can develop. Most are able to wean down on doses or medications or eventually stop them completely with time.

Communicate with your physician during this transition to give you guidance. If you are 100% plant based it is also important to take about 2500mcg of vitamin B12 once a week. You likely will start to feel more energy. The increased feeling of power may be related to the increased production and subsequent absorption of healthy neurotransmitters from the intestines to the brain. The more energy you have, the more motivated you will be to stick with your changes and add to it.

My wife, Joy, is a registered dietitian who teaches people how to eat a healthy whole food plant-based diet through her online program available at:

www.bringjoytoyourkitchen.com

She and I do want your eating to be joyful and make transformative changes to your health. Other resources and books are available to help you with recipes, expand your understanding of the science behind eating a plant-based diet, and other health benefits.

A simple checklist to track the servings during the day can be helpful, especially in your first 12 weeks. Check off each box for each daily serving.

Vegetables					

Leafy vegetables		

Fruit				

Legumes		

*Legumes are beans, peas, and lentils and are very important.

Whole cooked grains				

Nuts/seeds		

The daily dozen app by Dr. Greger also is a useful app to track your daily food intake and serve as a nice daily reminder. This can act as a good checklist, similar to a homework checklist a student may have to take home for homework, a "honey-do" list, and a grocery store list.

You may be thinking, "you only talk about a whole-foods plant-based diet, what about all the other diet options?" The most effective option is one that is predominantly a whole-foods plant-based diet. The more whole plant foods, the better you will do.

Chapter 12
Sleep and Fibromyalgia

Sleep has a powerful effect on how you feel. Remember the study where healthy college students developed FM in just three nights of deep sleep inhibition through loud noises startling them just as they were entering deep sleep. Unhealthy sleep can also occur through lousy sleep hygiene, also known as sleep habits. Good habits include the following:

- Go to bed and get up at the same time every day. Remember the activity monitor counting your steps. Now you can use it to track your sleep. Apps can be used on your phone that can track your sleep from your nightstand. The data can be eye-opening, showing a wide range of bedtimes and a lack of deep sleep or restless sleep.
- Get exercise regularly. This helps whether or not you have restless leg syndrome.
- Turn off electronics 1-2 hours before you go to bed.
- Limit your stress before bedtime.
- Avoid Caffeine and nicotine
- Avoid alcohol before bed. Many people self-medicate insomnia or RLS with alcohol. Unfortunately, this sabotages restorative sleep and can be addicting. It also has many other health consequences.
- Avoid naps, as this can make it hard to sleep later.
- Eating a diet with an abundant WFPBD (whole-foods plant-based diet) will significantly lower your risk of GERD (heartburn) and abdominal pains that could interrupt sleep. It also can reverse sleep apnea.

Sleep disorders you don't want to miss if you have FM:

1. **Restless Leg Syndrome.** RLS is a disorder caused by dysfunctions in dopamine levels. The textbook definition includes uncomfortable sensations in the legs, worsens as the night goes on, accompanied by an irresistible urge to move the legs, which temporarily improves with movement. RLS is usually due to an inherited deficiency in genes that regulate dopamine levels but can rarely be caused by low iron levels. The most common causes of low iron are poor absorption of iron from the intestines. The reduced absorption is most commonly related to celiac disease and Roux-en-Y gastric bypass surgery. Levels of iron can be measured through ferritin and serum iron. Other causes of low iron include blood loss. Relatively abrupt development of RLS symptoms should especially prompt evaluation for anemia from blood loss from such causes as a bleeding stomach ulcer. In children, RLS is often described as growing pains. Treatment with pramipexole, ropinirole, gabapentin, and pregabalin are beneficial for treatment. Treatment can calm the legs, which leads to uninterrupted sleep. High levels of exercise can sometimes eliminate the need for medications, but often medications are needed initially due to the profound fatigue from disrupted sleep with RLS.

2. **Obstructive sleep apnea (OSA).** Sleep can be disrupted hundreds of times a night, preventing one from getting into a deep sleep. This occurs when the back of the throat and tongue relaxes during sleep, causing the narrowing of the airway. The complete narrowing can occur, blocking the flow of vital oxygen to the body. Low levels of oxygen can cause the body to startle itself to restore airflow. Most often, people suffering from it are unaware unless their partner alerts them to snoring

and choking or gagging sounds they make throughout the night. OSA is diagnosed initially clinically through history and then confirmed with a sleep study that measures the number of obstructions during the night. Treatment with continuous air pressure known as CPAP or through adjustable air pressure known as auto pap are very effective. These are delivered through a mask and small machine and work by preventing the collapse of the back of the throat during sleep. Weight loss in overweight patients can eliminate the need for CPAP.

Chapter 13
Medications

Keep in mind that medications are one part of the solution in combination with education, understanding, and implementation of a healthy lifestyle of regular exercise, diet and sleep.

The most studied medications are tricyclic antidepressant (TCA) compounds. These work by blocking the reuptake of serotonin and norepinephrine reuptake, leading to increased levels. The most common and useful of these are cyclobenzaprine and amitriptyline. Tolerability can be a challenge with sedation, constipation, and dry mouth being common. These can be reduced by starting at a low dose and gradually increasing the amount until improvement in symptoms occurs, and secondary effects are minimized.

Selective serotonin acting medications such as citalopram and paroxetine don't work as well as they don't increase norepinephrine levels. Newer medications known as dual uptake inhibitors have proven to be much more beneficial. They increase the levels of both norepinephrine and serotonin. Duloxetine and milnacipran have been approved for the treatment of fibromyalgia. Venflexamine, although not explicitly approved for fibromyalgia, has shown benefit with nerve pain, tension headaches, and migraines, and mixed results for fibromyalgia.

The gain occurred regardless of whether someone was depressed. The most common secondary effects include stomach upset with some nausea and loose stools and cramping. These symptoms typically go away with time.

Starting at a lower dose for several days and then increasing minimize these issues, making them tolerable.

Alpha-2-delta ligands of voltage-gated calcium channels in the central nervous system, such as gabapentin and pregabalin, are effective in treating many different types of pain conditions, including fibromyalgia. Gabapentin was shown in several studies to be efficacious in FM. Pregabalin has demonstrated efficacy in three published trials and was approved for use in FM by the United States Food and Drug Administration (U.S. FDA) in 2007. These compounds may be better tolerated if a higher proportion of the dose (1200 to 2400mg/day of gabapentin or 300 to 450mg/day of pregabalin) is given at bedtime.

Take it about 2 hours before bedtime at a lower dose and adjust it until there is comfortable sleep without over sedation in the AM. If having pain issues during the day, daytime doses can be started but usually are about half the therapeutic nighttime dose.

Tizanidine is a centrally acting alpha-2 adrenergic agonist approved by the Food and Drug Administration to treat muscle spasticity associated with multiple sclerosis and stroke. Literature suggests that this agent is a useful adjunct in treating several chronic pain conditions, including chronic daily headaches and low back pain. A trial showed improvement in several parameters in FM, including sleep, pain, and measures of quality of life. It resulted in a reduction in substance P levels within the CSF of patients with fibromyalgia. The most common side effects of this class of drugs are lightheadedness, dizziness, edema, and weight gain.

Treatment with medications for restless leg syndrome, which commonly occurs with fibromyalgia, has also been shown to be effective in treating restless leg syndrome and improving fibromyalgia symptoms. These include pramipexole and ropinirole. These are effective when taken about 2 hours before bedtime. Infrequent side effects include unintentional gambling, likely from stimulating the dopamine reward center. The dose is adjusted to having a reversal of RLS symptoms without side effects.

Psychostimulant medications that treat ADHD can also be useful, as discussed earlier. They work to increase levels of dopamine and to some extent norepinephrine which tends to be at low levels. ADHD is ubiquitous in those with fibromyalgia but is often unrecognized. If ADHD is present, appropriate treatment reduces the catastrophization and improves filtering out distracting pain sensations. Most of the patients with untreated ADHD and fibromyalgia report feeling very overwhelmed. Organizing their day can be a challenge.

Untreated ADHD can lead to poor work performance and prolongation of the time needed to complete tasks. This inefficiency in completing tasks can lead to less time to exercise. Procrastination is common, so putting into action exercise, diet, and stress management plans can be significant barriers.

The first-tier medications described above are the first choices for medications to manage fibromyalgia. Second tier medications include tramadol. Tramadol is a medication that has the effect on 3 different receptors. This includes serotonin and norepinephrine and a weak effect on mu opioid receptors. The addictive potential is much lower than opioids.

Untreated ADHD also leads to "procrastineating." Instead of tackling the challenging project one might munch on calorie dense foods to get the dopamine. Untreated ADHD contributes to weight gain for many along with many other unhealthy consequences as discussed earlier.

What about opioids for FM management?

Studies show that opioids do not benefit those with FM. To the contrary they cause more harm in the long run. Observational studies show that those with opioid use have poorer outcomes than those treated with non-opioid medications that we have discussed earlier in the chapter. Despite the evidence, opioids are commonly used in clinical practice by many physicians for treating FM.

"Opioids get a lot of attention from both patients and physicians, and they distract from what we really should be doing to manage chronic pain," says Daniel Clauw, M.D., director of Michigan Medicine's Chronic Pain and Fatigue Research Center.

Opioids were a class of drugs that were never really shown to work for chronic pain and never really should have been used for chronic pain. Why don't opioids help? Don't they reduce pain? Many of you reading this book with FM may disagree feeling it has helped. "But if I miss a dose or try to reduce the dose, I feel worse. I can tell it helps me, Dr. Lenz." Let's look at the basic research on the likely reasons on why they are not effective.

You learned earlier that FM patients have lower levels of serotonin and norepinephrine in spinal fluid. Medications that increase these levels have been shown to be effective in treating FM. In contrast, the levels of natural opioids are higher in those with FM compared to those unaffected by FM. Earlier studies on levels of endorphins demonstrated no difference, but these studies were not able to reliably measure the levels.

issues that we talked about earlier including ADHD and Restless Leg Syndrome and then treating if present is important. The other preferred and approved medications for FM may be necessary along with lifestyle changes you have read about.

This isn't to excuse the addictions but understand them from a holistic perspective for you suffering with FM and possibly currently on opioids. The very medicine that may seem to be helping you, is actually limiting you from thriving with FM. Weaning off opioids should be done under careful supervision by your physician in conjunction with a comprehensive treatment with lifestyle and other appropriate medications.

"Jennifer" is a patient of mine who I met who got through her methadone use by such an approach. She had been an athlete when she was younger and into adulthood had been an active runner and worked out regularly at high levels into her adult life. She got married and had a son and worked at a local university helping with research.

She then went through a series of major stresses. She suffered the loss of her husband in a tragic farming accident. She came upon the horrific scene before the ambulance had arrived. She developed PTSD related to this event. In addition, she stopped exercising during her grieving and life transition. She then was in a minor car accident and had some whiplash. The whiplash persisted for months and required more regular doses of Vicodin to treat her pain as Tylenol and Motrin weren't effective.

Her pain spread to multiple areas of the body and only worsened with time. Her sleep was very poor with, unbeknownst to her, severe RLS. Her doctor had her go to the methadone clinic eventually as he didn't feel comfortable managing her chronic pain. She had been on methadone for a couple years when I met her.

I learned her story and evaluated her for FM which was positive. I also screened her for RLS and ADHD which also were positive. I discussed the relationships of FM, RLS, ADHD and what she was going through. I told her these could all be treated through a holistic comprehensive approach. She could get from just subsisting to living a fuller life. Treatment with gabapentin for her RLS reduced her pain. Treatment with Ritalin allowed her to complete tasks, focus, organize and plan her life, and feel much less overwhelmed.

She gradually became more and more active. She had fallen into the roller coaster of her activity varying from low to high levels. Proper pacing also reduced her pain levels. Her FIQ-R score dropped from a very high level to low to moderate levels. We talked about weaning off methadone which she was eager to do. Within a few months she weaned off methadone; and now was active, functioning, and living a life without the severe impairments she had when I first met her.

If all I did was tell her she needs to get off methadone and how unhelpful it was without identifying and treating the other comorbid issues, she would not have done well and would have been very frustrated.

Chapter 14
Stress Management

Stress is something that often happens to you where you may have limited control. As discussed earlier, experiencing traumatic events such as accidents, sexual assault, and combat atrocities can trigger FM-like syndromes in those who are more susceptible. Working with a therapist and treating comorbid conditions such as ADHD and anxiety may be necessary.

Having a supportive family to encourage you to stay on track with healthy lifestyle choices is valuable. This can include emotional support and practical support. Emotional support is having someone care about you and listen to your concerns. Practical help is someone who cooks a WFPB diet meal for you. It also includes offering to go for a walk with you after dinner or doing the dishes with you. Having an informed family member on what fibromyalgia is can help them work as an ally instead of a frustrated adversary.

Have fun together by scheduling enjoyable activities several times a week. Laughing helps us relax. Consider serving others as well by volunteering. Volunteering has many rewards and works by diverting attention from our pain to serving others. It reminds us that we have many valuable gifts and talents to assist others and helps us focus on what we can do and not what we can't do.

Avoid stress when possible. For many, watching the news on TV can add to a sense of feeling overwhelmed. Consider designating someone to filter the news for you to keep you informed on essential news.

Each person with FM and FM-like syndromes is unique, but there are many things shared with others. Partner with your physician and family to help navigate this once misunderstood syndrome. Thank you for taking the time to read this book, and I hope you found this edifying. I hope you are now much better informed, inspired, and equipped as you tackle FM.

Implementation intentions: examples of action and coping planning to specific barriers. Handling procrastination. If this is a consistent problem despite your best efforts, you may have ADHD. Get evaluated as treatment can make a big impact.

Apply problem solving. Keeping an exercise, activity, and diet journal can be a useful tool. Retrospective looks can teach you how your body reacts when you get out of a healthy routine. It also can give you confidence to manage your fibromyalgia.

Flare-up Management

Flare-ups are likely to occur for a variety of reasons. Some of these are in your control and some are out of your control. For example, intentionally planning a vacation starting with a flight at 6 AM and requiring you to wake at 3 AM can lead to a downward spiral for the rest of the week. Take a later flight that allows you to get your regular sleep. While waiting at the airport try to get up and go for a walk before the flight.

The approach will differ depending on the severity of the flare up. For mild flare ups, meticulous adherence to pacing your exercise and implementing healthy lifestyle choices may be all that is needed. For more severe episodes, restarting medications or increasing the dosages may be needed. This should be done through careful discussion with your physician.

Support from Family and Friends

Take good care of yourself. If you both fall overboard in the lake and are trying to survive, you first have to make sure you are safe and secure before you can help someone else struggling. Once you are secure with your life jacket on, you can safely rescue them as well. When you are in an airplane and the air pressure goes out, you have to grab oxygen for yourself before you can help someone else.

The same applies to managing FM. Keep on track with healthy lifestyle choices. You can benefit from the healthy choices making you even more resilient. Eating a WFPBD or going on a walk with your spouse would show support and the feeling that you are in it together.

It can be a challenge and walking a thin line in how you talk about FM with your spouse. Ideally your role isn't to be their doctor or accountability partner, but you can respectively inquire about how they are doing with their exercise and diet and what are ways for you to help.

Be positive. Living with FM can have its ups and downs and flare ups but keep looking to the positive and staying on track with their goals.

Fibromyalgia Log

Keeping track of key elements are important in long term management of your fibromyalgia. I want to put together what you can track. These include exercise, diet, sleep, stress, and medications. Linking these with your fibromyalgia score over the week are important. Dealing with fibromyalgia can be very emotional and overwhelming but logging these measures can help tie together a comprehensive cohesive approach from not just suffering and enduring fibromyalgia to one of thriving.

Exercise- Get an activity counter and count your steps.

Diet- Monitor your food intake and keep particular close attention to maximizing the food that contains fiber, whole-foods plant-based foods.

Sleep- Keep track of bedtime and wake times. Self-monitor for symptoms of RLS. If present bring it to the attention of your doctor. Apps on your smartphone can add a deeper level of sleep information including items such as how long it takes to fall asleep and when you wake up. It can give an indication of restless sleep as well. It can track the variation in sleep times from weekdays and workdays to weekends and your days off. If you have fibromyalgia, inconsistent sleep schedules add to stress.

Medications- Am I taking my medications as prescribed. What medications am I taking and why?

Dates Month- Days-	Steps	Diet	Bedtime	Wake time	Stress level 0-10	Medications
Monday						
Tuesday						
Wednesday						
Thursday						
Friday						

Made in the USA
Columbia, SC
23 July 2021